Respirato
Symptoms

T0092227

What Do I Do Now?: Palliative Care

SERIES EDITOR

Margaret L. Campbell, PhD, RN, FPCN
Professor Emeritus, Wayne University College of Nursing,
Detroit, MI

OTHER VOLUMES IN THE SERIES

Pediatric Palliative Care, Edited by Lindsay B. Ragsdale & Elissa G. Miller
Pain, Edited by Christopher M. Herndon

Respiratory Symptoms

Edited by

Margaret L. Campbell, PhD, RN, FPCN
Professor Emeritus, Wayne University College of Nursing,
Detroit, Michigan

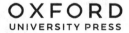

OXFORD
UNIVERSITY PRESS

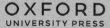

Oxford University Press is a department of the University of Oxford. It furthers
the University's objective of excellence in research, scholarship, and education
by publishing worldwide. Oxford is a registered trade mark of Oxford University
Press in the UK and certain other countries.

Published in the United States of America by Oxford University Press
198 Madison Avenue, New York, NY 10016, United States of America.

CIP data is on file at the Library of Congress
ISBN 978–0–19–009889–6

DOI: 10.1093/med/9780190098896.001.0001

Printed by Marquis Book Printing, Canada

Contents

List of Contributors   vii

Introduction   xi

1. **Dyspnea Assessment**   1
   Margaret L. Campbell

2. **Reducing Dyspnea by Optimizing Treatment of Chronic Obstructive Pulmonary Disease**   7
   Miranda Wilhelm and Jennifer Arnoldi

3. **Treating Chronic Breathlessness in Severe Chronic Obstructive Pulmonary Disease**   21
   Lynn F. Reinke, Mary M. Roberts, and Tracy A. Smith

4. **Dyspnea, Chronic Obstructive Pulmonary Disease, and Pulmonary Rehabilitation**   31
   DorAnne Donesky and Julie Howard

5. **Treating Episodic Breathlessness**   39
   Yvonne Eisenmann and Steffen Simon

6. **Reducing Episodic Dyspnea in Heart Failure**   49
   Beth B. Fahlberg and Ann S. Laramee

7. **Dyspnea in Pediatric Congenital Heart Disease**   61
   Jennifer Wright and Jessica L. Spruit

8. **Treating Chronic Dyspnea in Patients with Lung Cancer**   69
   Elizabeth A. Higgins, Susan Ezemenari, and Julia Arana West

9. **Treating Dyspnea Through Reducing Malignant Pleural Effusion**   77
   Christine A. Crader

10. **Treating Dyspnea in Lung Cancer with Noninvasive Ventilation**   87
    Vittoria Comellini and Stefano Nava

11. **Palliative Care for Infants with Bronchopulmonary Dysplasia**   95
    Christine A. Fortney and Jodi A. Ulloa

12. **Reducing Dyspnea by Treating Ascites**   101
    Habib A. Khan

13. **Panting for Breath in End-Stage Dementia**   109
    Hermien W. Goderie-Plomp, Carole Parsons, David R. Mehr,
    and Jenny T. van der Steen

14. **Last Days with Chronic Obstructive Pulmonary Disease**   119
    Margaret L. Campbell

15. **Withdrawal of Invasive Mechanical Ventilation**   125
    Margaret L. Campbell

16. **Palliative Sedation for Intractable Dyspnea**   135
    Patricia Bramati and Eduardo Bruera

17. **Sialorrhea in Amyotrophic Lateral Sclerosis**   145
    Mark B. Bromberg

18. **Death Rattle**   153
    Margaret L. Campbell

    Index   159

Contributors

Jennifer Arnoldi, PharmD, BCPS
Clinical Associate Professor
Southern Illinois University
Edwardsville (SIUE) School of
Pharmacy
Edwardsville, IL, USA

Patricia Bramati, MD
The University of Texas MD
Anderson Cancer Center
Houston, TX, USA

Mark B. Bromberg, MD, PhD
Department of Neurology
University of Utah
Salt Lake City, UT, USA

Eduardo Bruera, MD
The University of Texas MD
Anderson Cancer Center
Houston, TX, USA

**Margaret L. Campbell, PhD,
RN, FPCN**
Wayne State University, College
of Nursing
Detroit, MI, USA

Vittoria Comellini, MD
Respiratory and Critical Care Unit
University Hospital St.
Orsola-Malpighi
Bologna, Italy

Christine A. Crader, MD
Ascension Medical Group
Internal Medicine
Detroit, MI, USA

**DorAnne Donesky, PhD,
ANP-BC, ACHPN, ATSF**
Professor, School of Nursing
Touro University of California
Vallejo, CA, USA

Yvonne Eisenmann, MD
University of Cologne
Faculty of Medicine and
University Hospital
Department of Palliative
Medicine
Cologne, Germany

Susan Ezemenari, MD
Fellow, Palliative Medicine
Division of Internal Medicine,
Palliative Medicine and
Geriatrics
Medical University of South
Carolina
Charleston, SC, USA

Beth B. Fahlberg, PhD, MN, RN
University of Wisconsin
Madison, WI, USA

Christine A. Fortney, PhD, RN
Assistant Professor
The Ohio State University College
of Nursing
Martha S. Pitzer Center for
Women, Children and Youth
Columbus, OH, USA

**Hermien W. Goderie-Plomp,
MD, MSc, MSc**
Elderly Care and Palliative Care
Physician
De Zellingen, Rotterdam, The
Netherlands
Lecturer in Palliative Care
Leiden University Medical Center
Leiden, The Netherlands

Elizabeth A. Higgins, MD
Associate Professor of Internal
Medicine
Division of Internal Medicine,
Palliative Medicine and Geriatrics
Medical University of South Carolina
Charleston, SC, USA

Julie Howard, RRT, TTS, CCM
COPD Case Manager
Adventist Health Rideout
Marysville, CA, USA

Habib A. Khan, MD
Johns Hopkins Medicine
Department of Palliative Medicine
Wayne State University
Baltimore, MD, USA

**Ann S. Laramee, MS, ANP-BC,
ACNS-BC, CHFN, ACHPN,
FHFSA**
University of Vermont
Medical Center
Burlington, VT, USA

David R. Mehr, MD, MS
Professor Emeritus
Department of Family and
Community Medicine
University of Missouri
Columbia, MO, USA

Stefano Nava, MD
Department of Specialistic,
Diagnostic and Experimental
Medicine (DIMES), Alma
Mater Studiorum University
of Bologna
Bologna, Italy

**Carole Parsons, PhD,
MPharm, MPSNI**
Lecturer in Pharmacy Practice
School of Pharmacy
Queen's University Belfast
Belfast, UK

Lynn F. Reinke, PhD, RN
Claire Dumke Ryberg, RN
Presidential Endowed Chair in
End-of-Life/Palliative Care
University of Utah College of
Nursing
Salt Lake City, UT, USA

Mary M. Roberts, MSN, RN
Department of Respiratory
and Sleep Medicine, Westmead
Hospital
Ludwig Engel Centre for
Respiratory Research, Westmead
Institute for Medical Research
The University of Sydney at
Westmead Hospital
Westmead, New South Wales,
Australia

Steffen Simon, MD
Department of Palliative Medicine
University of Cologne
Faculty of Medicine and University
Hospital
Cologne, Germany

Tracy A. Smith, MD
Department of Respiratory and
Sleep Medicine, Westmead Hospital
The University of Sydney at
Westmead Hospital
Westmead, New South Wales,
Australia

Jessica L. Spruit, DNP, CPNP-AC
Pediatric Nurse Practitioner
Stepping Stones Pediatric Palliative
Care Program
University of Michigan
Health System
Ann Arbor, MI, USA

**Jodi A. Ulloa, DNP, APRN-CNP,
NNP-BC**
Assistant Professor of Clinical
Practice
The Ohio State University College
of Nursing
Martha S. Pitzer Center for
Women, Children and Youth
Columbus, OH, USA

**Jenny T. van der Steen, MSc,
PhD, FGSA**
Associate Professor
Leiden University Medical Center,
Department of Public Health and
Primary Care
Leiden, The Netherlands
Senior Researcher
Radboud University Medical
Center, Department of Primary
and Community Care
Nijmegen, The Netherlands

Julia Arana West, MD
Fellow, Palliative Medicine
Division of Internal Medicine,
Palliative Medicine and Geriatrics
Attending Physician, Department
of Emergency Medicine
Medical University of South
Carolina
Charleston, SC, USA

Miranda Wilhelm, PharmD
Clinical Associate Professor
Southern Illinois University
Edwardsville (SIUE) School of
Pharmacy
Edwardsville, IL, USA

Jennifer Wright, MS, CPNP
Stepping Stones Pediatric
Palliative Care
Michigan Medicine
Ann Arbor, MI, USA

Introduction

Margaret L. Campbell

In this volume, nearly all the chapters relate to the complex symptom dyspnea across diagnoses, lifespan, and care settings. Other chapters relate to oral and pharyngeal secretions. These topics are addressed from a palliative care context.

Dyspnea, also known as breathlessness, has been defined as a person's awareness of uncomfortable or distressing breathing. As this can only be known by the person, the term "respiratory distress" is used as the observed corollary relying on patient signs when the person is unable to report dyspnea, such as infants, young children, and adults with cognitive impairments, which may be acute or chronic.

Dyspnea develops when inspiratory effort, hypoxemia, and/or hypercarbia develops, which activates three redundant brain areas. In the cerebral cortex, the dyspneic person has an awareness of the change in breathing efficiency. The amygdala in the subcortical temporal lobe is activated when there is a threat to survival and produces a fear response. The pons in the brainstem reacts by activating compensatory accelerations of heart and respiratory rates and recruiting accessory muscles.

Assessment of dyspnea relies on self-report from as simple as a yes-or-no response to the query "Are you short of breath?" to more complex numeric scales (0–10) or categorical scales (none, mild, moderate, or severe). For patients unable to report dyspnea, observation scales such as the Respiratory Distress Observation Scale may be used. High-risk patients should be assessed at every clinical encounter.

Dyspnea is one of the most difficult symptoms to experience and is also one of the most difficult to treat, as the evidence base for this symptom lags behind other prevalent symptoms such as pain or nausea, to name two. Dyspnea is prevalent in patients with cardiopulmonary disorders and cancer, and it escalates as death approaches. The development of dyspnea in chronic disease is a predictor of mortality.

Dyspnea may be acute when a reversible etiology presents such as pneumonia, pleural effusion, or ascites. It is chronic in an irreversible condition such as chronic obstructive pulmonary disease (COPD), advanced heart failure, or congenital cardiac conditions. Episodic dyspnea may typify acute exacerbations in chronic conditions such as heart failure.

Treating dyspnea relies on a hierarchy of responses, beginning with treating underlying, reversible conditions such as infections, pleural effusions, volume overload, or ascites. Nonpharmacological treatments include pulmonary rehabilitation, noninvasive ventilation, balancing rest with activity, and optimal positioning. Pharmacological treatments include oxygen, bronchodilators, and opioids. In cases of refractory dyspnea, palliative sedation may be indicated.

Patients receiving invasive mechanical ventilation for respiratory failure may undergo ventilator withdrawal to afford a natural death. These patients are at very high risk for developing respiratory distress, which warrants careful attention to the processes to minimize distress.

Salivary secretions pose a significant problem for patients with bulbar-onset amyotrophic lateral sclerosis characterized by difficulties swallowing. Treatment begins with anticholinergic medications and may include botulinum toxin injections or irradiation of salivary glands.

Pharyngeal secretions, also known as death rattle, develops in about half of dying patients in the last days of life. Controversies about whether medications are indicated or effective make up the evidence base. Ethical concerns about medicating the patient to assuage the listener have been raised.

The contributors to this volume have addressed all the treatments currently known for dyspnea, respiratory distress, and secretions with a case study approach.

1 Dyspnea Assessment

Margaret L. Campbell

Stella is a nursing home resident in the advanced
stage of Alzheimer's disease. Her goals of care are
comfort-focused, with surrogate decisions previously
made to withhold tube feedings, intubation,
cardiopulmonary resuscitation, and hospitalization.
She sleeps most of the day and night and is
noncommunicative except for sounds of displeasure
such as when being bathed or turned. Stella is at high
risk for aspiration pneumonia; she is offered a soft,
easy-to-swallow diet with foods such as pudding,
scrambled eggs, oatmeal, and baby food.

On daily exam a change in her breathing is noted; it
is highly likely that Stella has developed pneumonia,
probably secondary to immobility or food or liquid
aspiration. The clinical team cannot elicit a dyspnea
assessment from Stella, and they know she is at risk
for respiratory distress.

What do I do now?

WHAT IS DYSPNEA?

Dyspnea is a person's awareness of uncomfortable or distressing breathing that can only be known by self-report. In symptom care a patient's self-report has long been held as the gold standard for assessment. In a palliative care context dyspnea should be assessed at every patient encounter, for example in the hospital whenever vital signs are obtained, or at every outpatient clinic visit, or at every house call for home-bound patients. Since dyspnea escalates as death nears, the frequency of assessment should be increased. Several tools are available for measuring and trending dyspnea that are appropriate in palliative care.

Unidimensional Assessment Tools

Responding to a symptom assessment requires several cognitive steps on the patient's part: (1) ascertain their sensation, (2) pay attention to the clinician's assessment instructions, (3) formulate a response, (4) communicate that response in some fashion, and (5) recall their previous report if trending is requested. When a patient is feeling poorly or is fatigued, these steps may pose difficulty and simpler tools are indicated.

The simplest measure is to ask for a "yes" or "no" response to the query "Are you short of breath?" or, in the case of the mechanically ventilated patient, "Are you getting enough air?" Knowing the presence or absence of dyspnea is helpful, but its intensity cannot be assessed with this approach. A more complex tool is a numeric rating scale, usually anchored at 0 for no dyspnea and 10 for the worst possible dyspnea. Patients may need guidance on how to use numbers to characterize their symptom intensity. A variation to using numbers is to ask for a categorical ranking (none, mild, moderate, severe). Some patients may find these categorical rankings easier to understand and relate to their experience than a numeric rating.

Another variation that can be used to rate intensity is a visual analog scale, typically a 100-mm scale anchored at 0 and 100, with tick marks at every 10 points (Figure 1.1). The patient points to a line on the scale representing their experience and the clinician can convert that to a numeric score; this approach is useful in the critical care setting with patients who are mechanically ventilated and nonverbal. A vertical scale was preferred by patients with chronic obstructive pulmonary disease (COPD).[1]

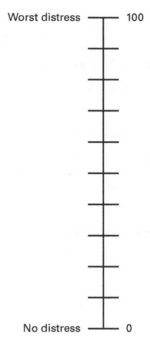

Worst distress ———— 100

No distress ———— 0

FIGURE 1.1. Visual analog scale for dyspnea

Multidimensional Assessment Tools

Dyspnea is a multidimensional symptom with physical and affective attributes that are not captured by the unidimensional tools just described. These scales may be applied by patients with intact cognition who may be receiving palliative care concurrently with disease treatment. The Dyspnea-12[2] is a multidimensional scale composed of 12 descriptors that are scored on a four-item scale with the points summed to produce a total dyspnea score (Table 1.1). Subscales for physical and affective domains can be derived. The focal point for this assessment is "these days," which captures the average experience of a chronic symptom.

The Multidimensional Profile (MDP)[3] comprises 11 numeric rating scales (0–10) of different sensory and affective breathlessness sensations and a "forced choice" item requiring respondents to select which of five sensory qualities best describes their breathlessness. Individual item ratings are reported, and subdomain scores can be calculated. Where a single score is sought by users, the MDP-A1 item (0–10 rating of breathlessness unpleasantness) was recommended by the developers; a total summed score of all items is not recommended for the MDP. The user specifies the focal event

TABLE 1.1. **The Dyspnea-12**

Item	None	Mild	Moderate	Severe
1. My breath does not go in all the way.				
2. My breathing requires more work.				
3. I feel short of breath.				
4. I have difficulty catching my breath.				
5. I cannot get enough air.				
6. My breathing is uncomfortable.				
7. My breathing is exhausting.				
8. My breathing makes me feel depressed.				
9. My breathing makes me feel miserable.				
10. My breathing is distressing.				
11. My breathing makes me agitated.				
12. My breathing is irritating.				

Reprinted with permission from J. Yorke.

(e.g., "after you climb three flights of stairs," "last minute of breathing on the mouthpiece") or timepoint (e.g., "right now") for the MDP, and can choose to use only one or a few of the instrument scales, depending on the clinical purpose of assessment. Permission for use must be obtained from the author.

The Modified Medical Research Council (MMRC) dyspnea scale[4] stratifies dyspnea into one of four scores relative to function, with 0 signifying dyspnea only with strenuous exercise and 4 representing too dyspneic to leave the house or dress. The MMRC dyspnea scale is best used to establish baseline functional impairment related to respiratory disease.

Observation Scale

Patients who are unable to provide a symptom report but can experience the symptom are vulnerable to over- or under-treatment. Respiratory distress is the observed corollary to reported dyspnea relying on patient signs. The Respiratory Distress Observation Scale[5] was developed for patients with advanced disease who are unable to self-report (Table 1.2). Eight variables are

TABLE 1.2. **Respiratory Distress Observation Scale**

Variable	0 points	1 point	2 points	Total
Heart rate per minute	<90 beats	90–109 beats	≥110 beats	
Respiratory rate per minute	≤18 breaths	19–30 breaths	>30 breaths	
Restlessness: non-purposeful movements	None	Occasional, slight movements	Frequent movements	
Accessory muscle use: rise in clavicle during inspiration	None	Slight rise	Pronounced rise	
Paradoxical breathing pattern	None		Present	
Grunting at end-expiration: guttural sound	None		Present	
Nasal flaring: involuntary movement of nares	None		Present	
Look of fear	None		Eyes wide open, facial muscles tense, brow furrowed, mouth open	

Source: m.campbell@wayne.edu

scored from 0 to 2 points and the points are summed to yield a total intensity score ranging from 0 to 16. Reliability and validity have been established across diagnoses and settings of care; intensity cut-points are 0–2 = no distress, 3 = mild distress, 4–6 = moderate distress, and 7 and higher = severe distress.[6,7]

SUMMARY

Several unidimensional and multidimensional scales and an observation scale were described as suitable for assessment in patients receiving palliative care. Selection of the optimal tool will depend on the patient's cognitive abilities, which are influenced by disease trajectory, fatigue, sedation, mechanical ventilation, and underlying conditions such as dementia.

Stella has a heart rate of 108 and respiratory rate of 22. She has slight restlessness and a slight rise in the clavicle, signifying accessory muscle use. There is no apparent paradoxical breathing, nor grunting, nor nasal flaring or a fearful facial expression. Thus, her RDOS score is 4, signifying moderate distress. The nurses elevated the head of her bed, placed a fan blowing on her cheek, and began immediate-release morphine elixir at 5 mg every 4 hours. Subsequent RDOS scores decreased to 2 or 3 with this regimen.

KEY POINTS TO REMEMBER

- Assessment is critical to optimizing treatment.
- Patient abilities will inform selection of an assessment tool or scale.
- Self-reported dyspnea presence and intensity is the gold standard.
- Respiratory distress signs are indicated for those who cannot report their experience.

References

1. Gift A. Validation of a vertical visual analogue scale as a measure of clinical dyspnea. *Rehab Nurs.* 1989;14:323–325.
2. Yorke J, Moosavi SH, Shuldham C, Jones PW. Quantification of dyspnoea using descriptors: development and initial testing of the Dyspnoea-12. *Thorax.* 2010;65(1):21–26.
3. Banzett RB, O'Donnell CR, Guilfoyle TE, et al. Multidimensional Dyspnea Profile: an instrument for clinical and laboratory research. *Eur Respir J.* 2015;45(6):1681–1691.
4. Mahler DA, Wells CK. Evaluation of clinical methods for rating dyspnea. *Chest.* 1988;93(3):580–586.
5. Campbell ML, Templin T, Walch J. A Respiratory Distress Observation Scale for patients unable to self-report dyspnea. *J Palliat Med.* 2010;13(3):285–290.
6. Campbell ML. Psychometric testing of a respiratory distress observation scale. *J Palliat Med.* 2008;11(1):44–50.
7. Campbell ML, Kero KK, Templin TN. Mild, moderate, and severe intensity cut-points for the Respiratory Distress Observation Scale. *Heart Lung.* 2017;46(1):14–17.

2 Reducing Dyspnea by Optimizing Treatment of Chronic Obstructive Pulmonary Disease

Miranda Wilhelm and Jennifer Arnoldi

JW, a 75-year old female, presents to the primary care clinic with a chief complaint of "This inhaler is not working." The patient reports shortness of breath with activities of daily living but has not experienced an exacerbation or hospitalization or used an oral corticosteroid related to chronic obstructive pulmonary disease (COPD) for the last year. Relevant medical history includes 60 pack-year history of smoking cigarettes (1 pack per day for 60 years; quit "cold turkey" approximately 1 year ago), COPD for 5 years, osteoporosis for 10 years, hypertension for 20 years, and rheumatoid arthritis for 33 years. Current medications include tiotropium HandiHaler, albuterol hydrofluoroalkane (HFA), salmeterol Diskus (recently added), alendronate, lisinopril/hydrochlorothiazide, methotrexate and hydroxychloroquine. Recent records indicate that her forced expiratory volume in 1 second (FEV_1) is 45% of predicted and her COPD Assessment Test (CAT) score is 18.

What do I do now?

The Global Initiative for Chronic Obstructive Lung Disease (GOLD) guidelines are updated and published on an annual basis. It is recommended that all healthcare providers incorporate this evidence-based guideline into their practice for the prevention, diagnosis, and treatment of COPD. Currently, the GOLD guidelines recommend short-acting bronchodilators, either a short-acting beta agonist (SABA) or a short-acting muscarinic antagonist (SAMA), for relief of acute symptoms in all patients. First-line maintenance pharmacotherapy includes the use of a long-acting bronchodilator such as a long-acting beta agonist (LABA) or a long-acting muscarinic antagonist (LAMA). Inhaled corticosteroids are considered the last option to reduce exacerbations (Table 2.1). It is important to continue these therapies through the end of life to manage symptoms and to maximize quality of life by minimizing dyspnea.

Selection of therapy for COPD should consider not only the patient's disease characteristics such as symptoms, exacerbation history, and future risks, but also their physical capabilities, cognitive function, and other comorbidities. The patient's previous experience with inhalation devices, their preferences, and insurance coverage of medication therapy should also be considered.

For established regimens, the patient's adherence and their inhaler technique should be assessed. If the patient is not using the inhaler as prescribed or their technique is poor, this could reduce the actual and perceived efficacy of the medication. Therefore, selecting the device can be just as important as selecting the appropriate class of medications to use in COPD. Four inhalation devices—metered-dose inhalers (MDIs), dry powder inhalers (DPIs), soft mist inhalers (SMIs), and nebulizers—are used in COPD pharmacotherapy. Table 2.2 lists their advantages and disadvantages.

INHALATION DEVICES

MDIs

MDIs consist of a canister, a metering chamber, and an actuator with a mouthpiece (Figure 2.1). The canister contains a solution of the medication and a propellant. Shaking the device disperses the propellant into the medication solution, creating the pressure needed for aerosolization. As the canister is depressed, the patient must be ready to inhale the dose. Thus,

TABLE 2.1. Inhaled Medications Commonly Used to Treat COPD

Pharmacological class	Generic drug name	Brand drug name	Inhalation type
Beta$_2$-agonists, short-acting (SABA)	Albuterol	Generics (various)	MDI, nebulization solution
		ProAir RespiClick (Teva)	DPI
		ProAir Digihaler (Teva)	DPI
		ProAir HFA (Teva)	MDI
		Proventil HFA (Merck)	MDI
		Ventolin HFA (GlaxoSmithKline)	MDI
	Levalbuterol	Generics (various)	Nebulization solution
		Xopenex HFA (Sunovion)	MDI
Beta$_2$-agonists, long-acting (LABA)	Arformoterol	Brovana (Sunovion)	Nebulization solution
	Formoterol	Perforomist (Mylan)	Nebulization solution
	Indacaterol	Arcapta Neohaler (Sunovion)	DPI, capsule-based dosage form
	Olodaterol	Striverdi Respimat (Boehringer Ingelheim)	SMI
	Salmeterol	Serevent Diskus (GlaxoSmithKline)	DPI
Anticholinergics, short-acting (SAMA)	Ipratropium	Generics (various)	Nebulization solution
		Atrovent HFA (Boehringer Ingelheim)	MDI

(*continued*)

TABLE 2.1. **Continued**

Pharmacological class	Generic drug name	Brand drug name	Inhalation type
Anticholinergics, long-acting (LAMA)	Aclidinium	Tudorza Pressair (Circassia)	DPI
	Glycopyrrolate	Seebri Neohaler (Sunovion)	DPI, capsule-based dosage form
		Lonhala Magnair (Sunovion)	Nebulization solution
	Revefenacin	Yupelri (Mylan)	Nebulization solution
	Tiotropium	Spiriva HandiHaler (Boehringer Ingelheim)	DPI, capsule-based dosage form
		Spiriva Respimat (Boehringer Ingelheim)	SMI
	Umeclidinium	Incruse Ellipta (GlaxoSmithKline)	DPI
Combination, SABA/SAMA	Albuterol/ ipratropium	Generics (various)	Nebulization solution
		Combivent Respimat (Boehringer Ingelheim)	SMI
Combination, LABA/LAMA	Formoterol/ aclidinium	Duaklir Pressair (Circassia)	DPI
	Formoterol/ glycopyrrolate	Bevespi Aerosphere (AstraZeneca)	MDI
	Indacaterol/ glycopyrrolate	Utibron Neohaler (Sunovion)	DPI, capsule-based dosage form
	Vilanterol/ umeclidinium	Anoro Ellipta (GlaxoSmithKline)	DPI

TABLE 2.1. **Continued**

Pharmacological class	Generic drug name	Brand drug name	Inhalation type
	Olodaterol/ tiotropium	Stiolto Respimat (Boehringer Ingelheim)	SMI
Combination, LABA/inhaled corticosteroid	Formoterol/ budesonide	Symbicort (AstraZeneca)	MDI
	Formoterol/ mometasone	Dulera (Merck)	MDI
	Salmeterol/ fluticasone	Advair HFA (GlaxoSmithKline)	MDI
		Advair Diskus (GlaxoSmithKline)	DPI
		AirDuo RespiClik (Teva)	DPI
		Wixela Inhub (Mylan)	DPI
	Vilanterol/ fluticasone	Breo Ellipta (GlaxoSmithKline)	DPI
Triple combination, LABA/LAMA/ inhaled corticosteroid	Vilanterol/ umeclidinium/ fluticasone	Trelegy Ellipta (GlaxoSmithKline)	DPI

MDI use requires hand–breath coordination, and conditions that can decrease dexterity (e.g., rheumatoid arthritis, Parkinson's disease) or cognitive performance may limit a patient's ability to accurately use the inhaler. Due to the propellant contained in MDIs, failure to coordinate breath with dose activation can result in medication being deposited in the mouth and/or throat or loss of drug into the air. Holding chamber/spacer devices, when combined with MDIs, may improve patient technique in terms of hand–breath coordination but still require some manual dexterity to manipulate and are bulky to handle.

TABLE 2.2. **Advantages and Disadvantages of Inhalation Devices**

Inhalation device	Advantages	Disadvantages
MDI	• Convenient/portable • Multidose devices • Short administration time • Counter indicates doses remaining	• Hand–breath coordination required • Multiple steps • Requires priming • Throat deposition, leading to adverse drug events
DPI	• Convenient/portable • Single-dose and multidose devices • Short administration time • Counter indicates doses remaining • Breath-actuated	• Requires moderate to high inspiratory flow rate • May require priming • Throat deposition, leading to adverse drug events
SMI	• Convenient/portable • Multidose devices • Short administration time • Counter indicates doses remaining	• Hand–breath coordination required • Requires assembly • Multiple steps • Requires priming
Jet nebulizer	• Hand–breath coordination not required • Minimal dexterity needed	• Temperature change of medication during use (cool) • Limited portability • Power source or battery pack needed • Requires assembly • Lengthy administration time (10–15 minutes) • Requires frequent cleaning • Not all medications available in this dosage form • Generates noise • Single dose

TABLE 2.2. **Continued**

Inhalation device	Advantages	Disadvantages
Ultrasonic nebulizer	• Portable • Quiet • Hand–breath coordination not required • Minimal dexterity needed	• Temperature change of medication during use (heat) • Power source or battery pack needed • Requires assembly • Administration time (5 minutes) • Requires frequent cleaning • Not all medications available in this dosage form • Single dose
Vibrating mesh nebulizer	• Portable • Quiet • Hand–breath coordination not required • Minimal dexterity needed • No temperature change of medication during use	• Expensive • Power source or battery pack needed • Requires assembly • Administration time (5 minutes) • Requires frequent cleaning • Not all medications available in this dosage form • Single dose

Asking the patient to demonstrate their technique with the inhaler may allow the provider to identify any potential errors in use that could prevent the medication from being effective. Common errors encountered in MDI use that could easily be identified through patient observation include failing to remove the device's mouthpiece cover before use; not sealing the mouth around the mouthpiece when actuating the dose; lack of coordination between activating the dose and inhaling; and inhaling via the nose rather than the mouth.

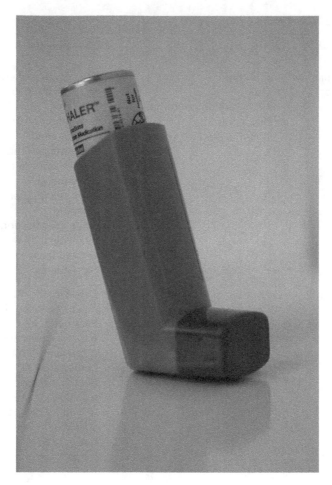

FIGURE 2.1. Metered-dose inhaler

Photo by Katherine Newman, PharmD.

DPIs

DPIs include a medication reservoir, an air inlet area, and a mouthpiece (Figures 2.2 and 2.3). The medication is in a dry powder dosage form that is drawn from the device using the patient's own breath. This may simplify the hand–breath coordination required by MDIs; however, the lack of propellant in these devices requires the patient to generate a sufficient inspiratory flow rate to inhale the entire dose of the medication. Patients

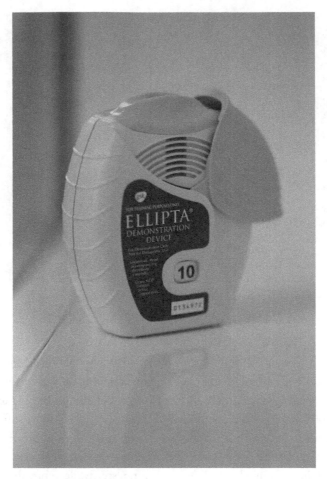

FIGURE 2.2. Dry powder inhaler: Ellipta

Photo by Katherine Newman, PharmD.

with advanced COPD may experience disease-related airflow limitation, leading to difficulties in taking a breath with sufficient force and volume to inhale the full dose of the medication. One complicating factor is that DPIs are manufactured with some degree of variability in design, including the turbulence and resistance of the product and device. Due to this, the patient's ability to use one type of DPI does not predict success with a DPI containing a different medication or administration device. A patient's peak

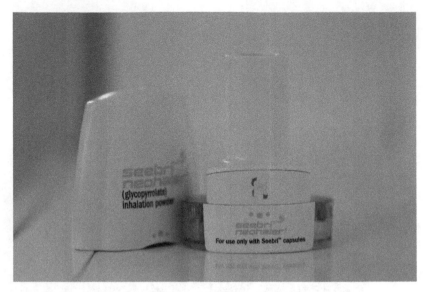

FIGURE 2.3. Dry powder inhaler: Neohaler

Photo by Katherine Newman, PharmD.

inspiratory flow rate (PIFR) can be obtained using a handheld inspiratory flow meter with an adjustable dial to simulate internal resistances of dry powder devices. For optimal DPI use, the patient should be able to attain at least 60 L/min; a PIFR less than 30 L/min is not likely to be sufficient.

All patients receiving a DPI should be educated to avoid breathing into the device or getting it wet. Each device contains unique instructions about breathing in (e.g., quickly and deeply; a long, steady, deep breath; inhaling deeply and forcefully; taking two breaths from the same dosage). Simple instructions could be given as "breathe in hard and fast." For DPIs, it is critical to consider the mechanism by which the dose is prepared for use; while the patient's breath is the driving force to disperse and deliver the medication, each device uses a different approach to allow this to happen. For some devices, the dose may be prepared by opening the mouthpiece cover with or without the need to activate an additional lever (e.g., Diskus, Ellipta). For others (e.g., HandiHaler, Neohaler), the patient needs to open a capsule from a blister pack, place the capsule into the device, and pierce the capsule before inhaling. These device differences should also be considered when selecting the device (i.e., whether the patient has the dexterity required to manipulate the capsule or the cognitive ability to follow dosing instructions) and when evaluating the patient's inhaler technique. Each step of the device's usage process creates the potential for user error.

Finally, patients using DPIs should be educated that once the dose has been prepared for inhalation they should not tip, shake, or otherwise disturb the contents inside the inhaler. If they do, they risk losing some of the medication prior to use.

SMIs

SMIs do not use a propellant; rather, a liquid formulation delivers medication as a fine mist aerosol for inhalation. The unique nozzle delivers medication at a slower velocity (1.5 seconds) compared to MDIs (100–400 milliseconds). SMIs were designed to make medication delivery easier than with MDIs, although some hand–breath coordination is still required. In addition, the devices require assembly before use, which may require some degree of manual dexterity and/or cognition (Figure 2.4).

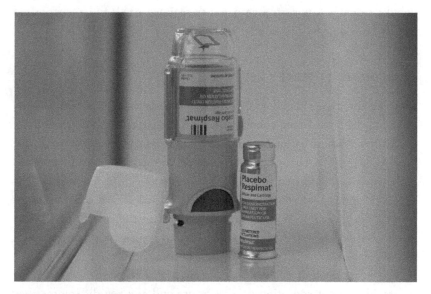

FIGURE 2.4. Soft mist inhaler

Photo by Katherine Newman, PharmD.

Nebulizers

Nebulizers turn liquid medication into an aerosol for inhalation. They offer an alternative to MDIs and DPIs for providing inhaled therapy to patients with COPD. Evidence suggests that the efficacy of nebulizer treatments in patients with COPD is similar to that with MDIs and DPIs. Several options are available for the type of nebulizer (e.g., jet, ultrasonic, and vibrating mesh). Nebulized medications eliminate the need for hand–breath coordination, but some dexterity may be needed to open the vial of liquid medication. Other considerations with nebulizer therapy include the possibility of longer treatment times compared to inhalation by MDIs, DPIs, or SMIs; portability of the nebulizer device selected; and the frequent cleaning required to maintain the device. Newer nebulizers have a shorter administration time (5–10 minutes vs. 15 minutes or more), use batteries rather than wall outlets, and are smaller in size to enhance portability. As COPD progresses and particularly at the end of life, patients may experience decreased PIFR, so use of handheld inhalers may become difficult. In this population, nebulized medication may offer improvement in symptom control and quality of life. Not every medication is available in nebulizer dosage forms, so each patient's regimen needs to be customized (see Table 2.1).

COMBINATION THERAPY REGIMENS

Once a patient's optimal device type has been identified and both the patient and the provider are comfortable with the patient's device technique, every effort should be made to continue the patient on the same device type when making changes to the inhaled regimen. For instance, if the patient has demonstrated proper technique with a tiotropium SMI (i.e., Spiriva Respimat) and the prescriber wishes to add a LABA for symptom control, switching to a combination olodaterol/tiotropium SMI (i.e., Stiolto Respimat) would allow the patient to use two medications with a single device to which they've already become accustomed. When it is necessary to switch device types or add an additional device, it is critical to provide patient education on device use and any key differences they should be aware of (e.g., using a slow, deep breath for the MDI vs. a quick, forceful breath for the DPI). Every effort should be made to verify the patient's understanding of the devices, optimally through use of demonstration and/or teach-back.

INHALER DEVICE TRAINING

The complexity of COPD regimens and devices and the likelihood of medication changes over the course of the chronic disease make comprehensive patient education of the utmost importance. Demonstrating inhaler technique, working with the patient until they can properly use the device, and using the teach-back method are crucial to prepare patients for safe and effective medication use. In addition, patients should regularly have their technique reviewed and receive additional education on any technique errors. Patients who are advanced in age and those who have cognitive impairment, complicated regimens, or multiple device types may require additional time and training in order to be successful. If available, devices such as the InCheck DIAL or the Vitalograph AIM (Aerosol Inhalation Monitor) may be used to assess the patient's inspiratory flow and appropriateness for a variety of devices. The InCheck includes the ability to simulate the resistance of a selected DPI to determine if the patient has an adequate inspiratory flow. The Vitalograph can be used with an attachment MDI or DPI simulator mouthpiece to analyze the patient's inhaler technique at various stages of the inhalation process, including breath-hold time at the end of the inhalation.

KEY POINTS TO REMEMBER

- Selection of therapy for COPD should consider not only the patient's disease characteristics but also their physical capabilities, cognitive function, and other comorbidities.
- Adherence and inhaler technique should be assessed prior to adding and/or changing pharmacotherapy.
- A variety of inhalation devices, including MDIs, DPIs, SMIs, and nebulizers, are available to individualize therapy, but these devices may require hand–breath coordination and/or dexterity so that the medication is administered correctly.

Further Reading

Ari A. Jet, ultrasonic, and mesh nebulizers: an evaluation of nebulizers for better clinical outcomes. *Eurasian J Pulmonol.* 2014;16:1–7.

Dal Negro RW. Dry powder inhalers and the right things to remember: a concept review. *Multidiscip Respir Med.* 2015;10(1):13.

Dhand R, Cavanaugh T, Skolnik N. Considerations for optimal inhaler device selection in chronic obstructive pulmonary disease. *Cleveland Clin J Med.* 2018;85(2 supp 1):S19–S27. doi:10.3949/ccjm.85.s1.04

GOLD Science Committee. Global Strategy for the Diagnosis, Management, and Prevention of Chronic Obstructive Lung Disease. https://goldcopd.org/wp-cont ent/uploads/2019/11/GOLD-2020-REPORT-ver1.1wms.pdf

Loh CH, Ohar JA. Personalization of device therapy: prime time for peak inspiratory flow rate. *Chronic Obstr Pulm Dis.* 2017;4(3):172–176. doi:10.15326/ jcopdf.4.3.2017.0155

Mahler DA. Peak inspiratory flow rate as a criterion for dry powder inhaler use in chronic obstructive pulmonary disease. *Ann Am Thorac Soc.* 2017;14(7):1103–1107. doi:https://doi.org/10.1513/AnnalsATS.201702-156PS

Rogliani P, Calzetta L, Coppola A, et al. Optimizing drug delivery in COPD: the role of inhaler devices. *Respir Med.* 2017;124:6–14.

Tashkin DP. A review of nebulized drug delivery in COPD. *Int J Chron Obstruct Pulmon Dis.* 2016;11:2585–2596.

3 Treating Chronic Breathlessness in Severe Chronic Obstructive Pulmonary Disease

Lynn F. Reinke, Mary M. Roberts, and Tracy A. Smith

Mr. B is a 72-year-old man with severe chronic obstructive pulmonary disease (COPD) on 2 liters per minute (LPM) of supplemental oxygen therapy continuously. Past medical history: congestive heart failure, anorexia, and anxiety. He presented to the emergency department twice last year for COPD exacerbations and was admitted to the hospital once, requiring bilevel ventilation. Today, at the clinic, he is alert and frail and has a body mass index (BMI) of 17 kg/m^2. At rest he can speak in full sentences; however, ambulating 25 feet induces breathlessness. On a scale from 1 to 10 (1 = no dyspnea, 10 = severe dyspnea) he rates his dyspnea at rest as 5, and on exertion as 8. Physical exam findings: barrel-chested, decreased breath sounds with mild crackles at bilateral bases. His wife of 50 years is his primary caregiver and assists with daily care, including bathing, dressing, medications, and meal preparation.

What do I do now?

CLINICAL PROBLEM: OVERVIEW OF COPD AND DYSPNEA

Worldwide, COPD currently ranks seventh as the cause of years of life lost, sixth as the cause of years living with disability for women, and ninth as the cause of years living with disability for men. Dyspnea, also known as breathlessness, affects 56–98% of patients with advanced COPD, and it impacts every aspect of their lives. Often patients live with breathlessness for years.

The American Thoracic Society (ATS) defines dyspnea as a subjective experience of breathing discomfort that comprises qualitatively distinct sensations that vary in intensity. The experience derives from interactions among multiple physiological, psychological, social, and environmental factors and may induce secondary physiological and behavioral responses.

Like all symptoms, breathlessness is a complex phenomenon that may be impacted by a number of interrelated issues, such as anxiety, depression, culture, previous experiences, and comorbidity. Breathlessness-related anticipatory fear and anxiety has recently been shown to exacerbate the experience. Breathlessness may occur during exertion or at rest, and it increases during exacerbations. Patients may be unable to walk small distances and can even get breathless with toileting.

PHYSIOLOGY OF BREATHLESSNESS

COPD is characterized by obstructive spirometry following the administration of a bronchodilator. While spirometry, in part, delineates severity in COPD, some people with relatively preserved spirometry will describe significant breathlessness, while some with physiologically advanced disease do not describe the symptom.

Breathlessness may be thought of as an imbalance between the demand to breathe and the ability to respond to this demand, sometimes called neuromechanical/neuroventilatory dissociation. Essentially, the respiratory center in the brainstem determines what respiration is required to meet the current physiological needs. This requirement is communicated to the respiratory system and to higher centers in the brain. When the respiratory system is unable to match the requirements, breathlessness ensues.

In COPD, the predominant problem leading to breathlessness is reduced inspiratory capacity. This occurs as bronchial obstruction and/or pulmonary emphysema, leading to "gas trapping" inside the lung. This reduces the space available for inspiration. Importantly, this "trapped gas" does not contribute to the exchange of oxygen and carbon dioxide. Exertion induces dynamic hyperinflation, leading to worse gas trapping and further compromising inspiratory capacity, as well as contributing to the development of hypoxemia and hypercarbia. When inspiratory capacity is less than the required tidal volume, breathlessness ensues. To experience this, try the following experiment: Find a set of stairs; breathe in; breathe in a little more; breathe out just that last little bit; try walking up the stairs just breathing in and out that last little bit without letting go of the first breath you took in. Other factors, such as poor gas exchange, skeletal/respiratory muscle weakness, and muscular fatigability, also contribute.

PSYCHOSOCIAL NEEDS

Living with advanced COPD often has psychological consequences and engenders high social support needs. For example, symptoms of depression are reported by 17–77% of patients and anxiety is reported by 32–57%. Breathlessness and anxiety are closely related. Anxiety is an emotional response to breathlessness and in turn increases the perception of breathlessness (Figure 3.1). Patients may fear death and suffocation. Distress and panic during the night are frequently experienced, resulting in sleep disturbance. Both anxiety and depression result in considerable burden and impaired quality of life but are also associated with a worse survival prognosis. Nevertheless, recognition of anxiety and depression is often limited, so screening for these symptoms is important. It is enormously reassuring for patients to learn that they are very unlikely to die during an acute episode of breathlessness, and that most people who die of COPD do so comfortably, without significant breathlessness.

The high daily symptom burden, physical limitations, and care dependency may result in social isolation, as well as a change in social role. Some patients feel ashamed of their symptoms (such as coughing) and the treatments they require (such as supplemental oxygen or an inhaler), while others may feel stigma related to current or previous behaviors that may be illness-related (such as smoking). As the disease progresses, patients

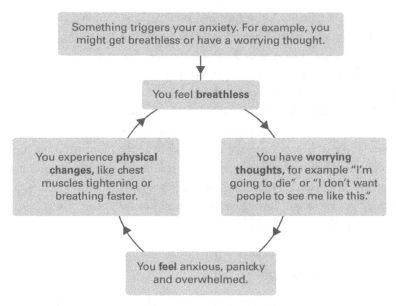

FIGURE 3.1. The dyspnea/anxiety cycle

become more restricted in their activities, including hobbies and socializing. Although these social consequences of the disease are of major importance to patients, they are often ignored by clinicians. Patients' spiritual needs are also often overlooked. Approximately 90% of patients with advanced COPD reported that their clinician didn't ask about their spiritual or religious beliefs. Patients may experience loss of hope and dreams. Finding ways to bring meaning into their lives and/or making referrals to chaplaincy or patients' religious leaders may help ease distress.

NONPHARMACOLOGICAL INTERVENTIONS FOR BREATHLESSNESS

As the pathophysiology of chronic breathlessness is complex and multidimensional, its treatment is similarly complex and multidimensional. When treating chronic breathlessness, a comprehensive assessment of the patient must be undertaken, and all reversible issues must be addressed and comorbidities maximally treated. If breathlessness remains, there are many nonpharmacological interventions that can be tried to address it (Box 3.1).

Pulmonary Rehabilitation and Physical Activity

Breathlessness may lead to avoidance of activity, resulting in deconditioning and increased symptom experience. Pulmonary rehabilitation (PR) reduces breathlessness and ameliorates deconditioning; however, some patients decline to participate, citing breathlessness. Encouraging a simple increase in physical activity may be the first step. Getting patients to try a pedometer may encourage increased physical activity, potentially leading to increased confidence to accept enrollment in PR.

Positioning and Breathing Techniques

Showing patients different positions and breathing techniques gives them tools to manage their breathlessness and gain some control. Mr. B and his wife should be taught these techniques so that she can encourage and guide him to try these when he is experiencing breathlessness at rest and during exertion. Such techniques include the *lean-forward position, pursed-lip breathing, controlled breathing,* and *recovery breathing.*

By adopting a lean-forward position, which passively fixes the shoulder girdle, patients effectively increase the efficiency of the diaphragm by improving the length–tension state, diminishing breathlessness. Encouraging Mr. B to also drop his shoulders will allow the accessory muscles to work more efficiently.

Other simple breathing techniques, such as pursed-lip breathing ("smell the roses, flicker the candle") and controlled breathing (normal tidal breathing, moving the stomach out during inhalation with relaxed shoulders and upper chest), can decrease breathlessness and give patients a sense of control. Controlled breathing promotes efficient breathing and use of accessory muscles, but regular practice is required. Mr. B needs to be encouraged to practice this technique when he is not breathless so that he can master the skill.

Recovery breathing (concentrating on the "breath out," gradually increasing in duration to prevent/reverse dynamic hyperinflation) can be taught by recommending that the patient "breathe around the rectangle," using the short side of the rectangle to guide the "in breath" and the longer sides to guide the "out breath." Visualizing a rectangle also helps distract the patient from the uncomfortable sensation of breathlessness. Encouraging Mr. B to look for a rectangular shape to focus on when he is breathless can assist with mastering recovery breathing.

Handheld Fans

Using a handheld fan directed at the lower half of the face can reduce the sensation of breathlessness. Handheld fans are a simple, cheap intervention that give patients a sense of control over their breathlessness. Giving Mrs. B the task of getting the fan during an attack can also give her the sense that she can assist with treatment. Patients and caregivers may think a fan is a "gimmick," so a brief explanation of the evidence and mode of action may encourage usage. Handheld fans vary in quality (airflow, noise, ease of use), so demonstrating and/or providing a high-quality fan is important. A tabletop fan near the patient may be useful when the patient becomes too weak to hold the small fan.

Energy Conservation

Energy conservation techniques enable people to participate in both essential activities (such as self-care activities) and leisure pursuits that promote social interaction, meaning, and enjoyment. Such techniques include sitting to perform activities often associated with standing (such as showering and cooking) and using aids.

Wheeled walking aids reduce breathlessness and increase walking distance by utilizing the lean-forward position for ambulating. Many walking aids incorporate a seat to enable rest if needed. Patients may resist using walking aids for a variety of reasons, but, once again, explaining the mode of action may help. Many patients find that a shopping cart provides similar support to a wheeled walker; encouraging patients to try a shopping cart on their next outing also may be helpful.

Other nonpharmacological interventions have been shown to reduce breathlessness but are less easily adopted into clinical practice (chest wall vibration, neuromuscular electrical stimulation) or have a lower evidence base (cognitive-behavioral therapy, relaxation, acupuncture).

PHARMACOLOGICAL MANAGEMENT OF BREATHLESSNESS

A variety of pharmacological approaches have been used. As in all areas of clinical care, all nonpharmacological interventions should be exhausted before pharmacological methods are added. Of particular relevance to COPD, patients should complete PR, preferably within the last 12 months, as the benefits of rehabilitation may wane after a year. Additionally, patients with severe COPD should receive maximally tolerated inhaled therapy, instructions on how to use an inhaler, and regular review to ensure correct inhaler technique. Long-term oral steroids have no role in reducing breathlessness.

Systemic Opioid Therapy

Opioids, particularly low-dose morphine (<30 mg/day), have the most evidence for efficacy for breathlessness. Constipation often occurs with opioid therapy at any dose, and laxatives should be prescribed concomitantly. While more serious side effects are rare, the literature is divided as to whether there may be long-term mortality impacts. Due consideration should be given to medication intolerances and other clinical considerations, particularly renal function. Patients and families may have concerns about initiating opioids; an open discussion regarding the goals of therapy and any concerns they may have is recommended. Opioids would be appropriate for Mr. B if nonpharmacological therapy is insufficiently effective. Start at a small dose (for instance, 10 mg/day) and increase to a maximum of 30 mg/day, depending on efficacy and side effects.

Benzodiazepines

This class of medication is sometimes used to relieve breathlessness; however, evidence suggests poor efficacy, significant side effects (falls, fractures,

COPD exacerbations, pneumonia, dementia, pancreatitis, cancer), and increased mortality. Given the limited evidence of benefit and documented risk of harms, careful, individualized consideration should be made before prescribing these agents for breathlessness.

Other Therapies

A range of other therapies have been trialed with limited evidence of efficacy and/or a limited literature base. Oral N-acetylcysteine, mirtazapine, and theophylline have been trialed but require further investigation. There are physiological reasons to consider nebulized opioids or nebulized furosemide; however, again, more research is needed. As yet, there is no research to support the use of cannabinoids. While patients, and some health professionals, often believe oxygen ameliorates breathlessness, there is little evidence to support this claim unless hypoxia is present.

MANAGEMENT OF ACUTE EPISODES OF BREATHLESSNESS

"Dyspnea crisis" is defined as a "sustained and severe resting breathing discomfort that occurs in patients with advanced, often life-limiting illness and overwhelms the patient and caregivers' ability to achieve symptom relief." Dyspnea crisis usually occurs in patients with underlying chronic breathlessness and may result in overutilization of healthcare resources. Management requires an individualized approach, focused on prevention of episodes, early identification and management of exacerbations, and judicious use of hospitalizations. The ATS statement provides a mnemonic, COMFORT, that caregivers can use to remember the steps for managing a dyspnea crisis:

Call for help.
Observe the degree of respiratory difficulty.
Medications such as inhaled bronchodilators or morphine may help.
Fan to create air movement.
Oxygen can be administered or increased.
Reassure.
Take your time.

Simpler interventions include the 3 F's (Fan, lean Forward, and Focus on the out breath) and the 3 P's (Pause, Position [lean forward], and Purse lips).

BREATHLESSNESS SERVICES

An integrated way of assisting patients with chronic breathlessness has recently emerged: holistic breathlessness services that combine respiratory and palliative care. While such services are not universal, a recent systematic review examined a number of randomized controlled trials investigating the use of multidisciplinary teams to address breathlessness. Overall, these services were found to have a positive impact on breathlessness and were highly valued by patients and their loved ones.

Now back to Mr. B. He and his wife have learned various approaches to help outsmart his breathlessness. Now when he experiences a breathlessness episode, instead of becoming panicked he uses his handheld fan, leans slightly forward, and begins pursed-lip breathing and/or "breathing around the rectangle." If this doesn't help after 5 minutes, he tries his short-acting bronchodilator. Mr. B uses recovery breathing (breathing around the rectangle) during exertion, and he ambulates with a rollator. He conserves energy by using a terrycloth bathrobe to dry off after showering instead of toweling himself dry, and he sits on a shower stool to shave, groom, and shower. He enjoys sitting in his yard or at a window watching birds at the feeder and interacts with his grandchildren online. He goes to PR twice a week.

KEY POINTS TO REMEMBER

- Altered respiratory mechanics pathognomonic to COPD drive breathlessness.
- Nonpharmacological interventions, particularly when delivered by a multidisciplinary team, frequently improve breathlessness so well that no further measures are required.
- If medications are required, oral long-acting opioids, particularly morphine, have the best evidence for efficacy and safety.

Further Reading

Abdallah SJ, Jensen D, Lewthwaite H. Updates in opioid and nonopioid treatment for chronic breathlessness. *Curr Opin Support Palliat Care*. 2019;13(3):167–173.

Booth S, Burkin J, Moffat C, Spathis A, eds. *Managing Breathlessness in Clinical Practice*. Springer; 2014.

Brighton LJ, Miller S, Farquhar M, et al. Holistic services for people with advanced disease and chronic breathlessness: a systematic review and meta-analysis. *Thorax*. 2019;74(3):270.

Janssen DJ, Spruit MA, Leue C, et al. Symptoms of anxiety and depression in COPD patients entering pulmonary rehabilitation. *Chron Respir Dis*. 2010;7(3):147–157.

Johnson M, Barbetta C, Currow D, et al. Management of chronic breathlessness. In: Bausewein C, Currow D, Johnson M, eds. *Palliative Care in Respiratory Disease*. ERS monograph 73. European Respiratory Society; 2016: 19.

Luckett T, Phillips J, Johnson MJ, et al. Contributions of a hand-held fan to self-management of chronic breathlessness. *Eur Respir J*. 2017;50(2):1700262.

Mularski RA, Reinke LF, Carrieri-Kohlman V, et al. An official American Thoracic Society workshop report: assessment and palliative management of dyspnea crisis. *Ann Am Thorac Soc*. 2013;10(5):S98–S106.

O'Donnell DE, Webb KA, Harle I, Neder JA. Pharmacological management of breathlessness in COPD: recent advances and hopes for the future. *Expert Rev Respir Med*. 2016;10(7):823–834.

Parshall MB, Schwartzstein RM, Adams L, et al. An official American Thoracic Society statement: update on the mechanisms, assessment, and management of dyspnea. *Am J Respir Crit Care Med*. 2012;185(4):435–452.

Qaseem A, Wilt TJ, Weinberger SE, et al. Diagnosis and management of stable chronic obstructive pulmonary disease: a clinical practice guideline update from the American College of Physicians, American College of Chest Physicians, American Thoracic Society, and European Respiratory Society. *Ann Intern Med*. 2011;155(3):179–191.

4 Dyspnea, Chronic Obstructive Pulmonary Disease, and Pulmonary Rehabilitation

DorAnne Donesky and Julie Howard

Dr. Timothy Smith, a wheelchair-bound 74-year-old man has severe chronic obstructive pulmonary disease (COPD) with air trapping.

He has been selected by his previous university to receive a lifetime achievement award for his cutting-edge contributions to his field, and he would like to walk from his chair to the stage and back when he receives this award. Currently, he is able to walk a maximum of 30 feet with a walker around his home; otherwise, he requires a wheelchair whenever he leaves the home because of severe dyspnea with minimal exertion.

Assessment reveals a cachectic elderly gentleman using 3 liters per minute of continuous oxygen with e-tanks attached to the wheelchair and an oxygen saturation of 92% at rest. Six-minute walk was terminated after 40 feet due to dyspnea. Uses accessory muscles with quiet breathing. Lungs: Increased anteroposterior diameter, clear but diminished lung sounds. No peripheral edema. He has no other comorbidities.

What do I do now?

This patient is on maximum therapy for his severe COPD according to the Global Initiative for Chronic Obstructive Lung Disease (GOLD) guidelines.[1,2] His dyspnea, worsened by hyperinflation, is limiting his activities.[3] It is unclear whether his limitations on the 6-minute walk are related to lung impairment alone, or whether enhanced conditioning and symptom management strategies might provide functional improvement. His physiological testing results might indicate that he is unlikely to meet this goal, but outliers occur frequently enough that it is worthwhile to offer him a graduated pulmonary conditioning treatment plan that begins with minimal exertion and see if he can tolerate slight increases in exercise over time; he is anxious and also highly motivated. He needs to improve his confidence, decrease his anxiety, and ensure he has the strength and endurance to walk the distance required to receive his award.

The Breathing, Thinking, Functioning (BTF) Model developed by the Cambridge Breathlessness Intervention Service[4] provides guidance for addressing the dyspnea of a patient in this condition (Figure 4.1). All three

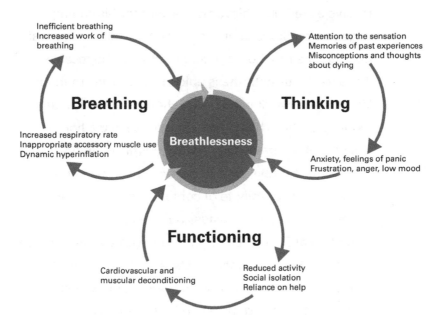

FIGURE 4.1. The Breathing, Thinking, Functioning Model

Reproduced with permission of the Cambridge Breathlessness Intervention Service[4] (email communication from Anna Spathis, November 11, 2019)

sections of the model apply to this patient, and the clinician must prioritize and address one section at a time. Dr. Smith is deconditioned, as specified by the Functioning section of the model; his hyperinflation might be improved with attention to the Breathing section; and his anxiety and panic may be addressed by the Thinking section.

Given that Dr. Smith's primary motivation is to walk across the stage to receive his award, the Functioning section of the model is the best place to begin his treatment plan. Pulmonary rehabilitation is a comprehensive intervention that includes exercise training, education, and support for patients with chronic lung disease to optimize their functioning and quality of life.[5,6] Although he was dubious and didn't think it would help, Dr. Smith agreed to try the recumbent stepper and recumbent stationery bicycle with minimal resistance on both for a goal of 3–5 minutes each and a 10-minute rest in between sets. His initial exercise sessions were individual 1:1 sessions with a respiratory therapist. On the first day, after arriving in a wheelchair, he was only able to do 2 minutes on the recumbent stepper. After resting for 7 minutes, he was able to do 3 minutes on the recumbent stationery bicycle. His oxygen saturation fell to 87% with exercise, so his liter flow was increased to 4 liters per minute with exercise. He declined any further endurance exercise that day but was willing to use 1-lb hand weights to do some upper body strengthening exercises. At the end of the first day, he was able to do some seated post-exercise stretches. He was very tired at the end of the first day and so additional education was not offered.

Dr. Smith's pulmonary rehabilitation program was scheduled three times a week, and when he returned for the second session, he reported surprise that he felt good, although his muscles were fatigued the day after his first session. Now, he was ready and guardedly enthusiastic to try his second exercise session. This time, he turned up his oxygen to 4 liters per minute prior to the start of exercise, and was able to do two repetitions on the recumbent bike, once again for 3 minutes each, with a 7-minute rest between the two repetitions. He was also able to tolerate 3 minutes on the recumbent stepper, upper body strengthening with 1-lb weights, and post-exercise upper body stretching while seated in his wheelchair.

While he was exercising, the respiratory therapist noticed a very shallow and rapid breathing pattern, consistent with the Breathing section of the

BTF Model. Prior to the second repetition, she demonstrated pursed-lip breathing while coordinating the pace of breathing with his movements, with a short inhale and a longer exhale. For the remainder of his exercise, she coached him to practice this breathing technique.

After 2 weeks (six sessions) of 1:1 exercise, Dr. Smith had progressed to the point where he and the therapist agreed that he was ready to join a small pulmonary rehabilitation group. By this point, he knew how to use the exercise equipment, and although his exercise prescription was still limited, he knew how to pace himself and do multiple repetitions after brief rest periods. According to the BTF Model, social isolation is a significant factor caused by breathlessness and reduced functioning. Offering Dr. Smith an opportunity to meet other pulmonary rehabilitation participants would give him "vicarious experiences" of observing others with the disease who have been able to reduce their dyspnea and enhance their functioning through exercise.[7] It also gave him the opportunity to socialize with others who use oxygen and share similar physical limitations.

One month after starting the rehabilitation program, Dr. Smith asked to try the treadmill with a therapist standing next to him. Initially he started at 0.5 mph for 5 minutes, but given the conditioning he had already been doing on the recumbent bicycle and stepper, he was able to progress faster on the treadmill—up to 0.7 mph for 10 minutes by the following week, in addition to his stepper and bicycle routine. After 2 months, Dr. Smith walked into the pulmonary rehabilitation department, using a walker. The others in the group gathered around and offered him congratulations and accolades. By this point, he was able to do 30 minutes of endurance exercise split between the three modes of exercise, and he used 3-lb hand weights for the strengthening exercises with the group. He was also able to stand for the pre- and post-exercise flexibility and balance exercises.

Over the second month, the respiratory therapist continued to teach him breathing strategies to increase the efficiency of his breathing and decrease the work of breathing.[8] In addition to pursed-lip breathing and pacing his breath, she taught him to focus on the subtle upward-and-outward movement of his lower ribs (similar to the movement of a bucket handle being raised) to enhance the change in volume and movement of air during the respiratory cycle, and allow gentle spinal movements up with inhalation and relaxed with exhalation.

The pulmonary rehabilitation class included educational sessions where Dr. Smith was taught about his medications, proper inhaler use, the importance of notifying his clinician at the first sign of an exacerbation, optimal nutrition, and energy conservation.[5] During the course of the rehabilitation class, he began to recognize that his chronic dyspnea was not dangerous,[9] and that avoiding it was actually leading him to be more dyspneic because of deconditioning. His conversations with the others in the class helped him normalize his sensations of dyspnea and panic, and he began to realize that he could live comfortably with some degree of dyspnea—the concern was when it overwhelmed his ability to cope with it.[10] He began to develop new ways of thinking about his symptoms and illness, which decreased the panic and anxiety that had previously overwhelmed him at times.[11]

By the time that the rehabilitation program concluded 3 months later, Dr. Smith was still walking with a walker. However, he continued to exercise on his own and a month later, when he walked across the stage to receive his reward, he was able to do so with only the help of a cane. He called to let the rehabilitation therapist know of his success. He joined a group of pulmonary rehabilitation graduates who met once a month for coffee at a local restaurant and maintained those friendships for at least a year after he graduated from rehabilitation.

KEY POINTS TO REMEMBER

- In people with COPD, their chronic dyspnea is never dangerous. Although they feel afraid to increase their shortness of breath by exerting themselves, exercise is actually the best thing they can do to increase their tolerance for daily activities. If exercise were a pill, it would be malpractice not to prescribe it for people with COPD!
- Dyspnea in people with COPD is caused by deconditioning as well as lung disease. Paradoxically, increased regular exercise will decrease dyspnea over time as the person becomes more conditioned.
- Anybody can exercise, regardless of severity of lung disease. Use baby steps to start very slowly and briefly and increase

intensity and duration very gradually—a few seconds more each day and a few steps more each session.

- Anyone who is short of breath will likely be anxious. Normalize it, and help them find the level of dyspnea they can tolerate while exercising. Customize their exercise program based on what they can tolerate and update their exercise prescription every session.
- If you don't have pulmonary rehabilitation available in your community, partner with outpatient physical therapy, a local gym that caters to older adults, and the lung association to provide exercise and support.
- Dyspnea is multifactorial—the Breathing, Thinking, Functioning Model provides guidance for evaluation and treatment priorities.

References

1. Gupta N, Agrawal S, Chakrabarti S, Ish P. COPD 2020 guidelines—what is new and why? *Adv Respir Med.* 2020;88(1):38–40.
2. GOLD Science Committee. 2020. Global Strategy for the Diagnosis, Management, and Prevention of Chronic Obstructive Pulmonary Disease. www.goldcopd.org
3. O'Donnell DE, Milne KM, James MD, de Torres JP, Neder JA. Dyspnea in COPD: new mechanistic insights and management implications. *Adv Ther.* 2020;37(1):41–60.
4. Spathis A, Booth S, Moffat C, et al. The Breathing, Thinking, Functioning clinical model: a proposal to facilitate evidence-based breathlessness management in chronic respiratory disease. *NPJ Prim Care Respir Med.* 2017;27(1):27.
5. Spruit MA, Singh SJ, Garvey C, et al. An official American Thoracic Society/European Respiratory Society statement: key concepts and advances in pulmonary rehabilitation. *Am J Respir Crit Care Med.* 2013;188(8):e13–64.
6. McCarthy B, Casey D, Devane D, Murphy K, Murphy E, Lacasse Y. Pulmonary rehabilitation for chronic obstructive pulmonary disease. *Cochrane Database Syst Rev.* 2015(2):CD003793.
7. Selzler AM, Rodgers WM, Berry TR, Stickland MK. Coping versus mastery modeling intervention to enhance self-efficacy for exercise in patients with COPD. *Behav Med.* 2020;46(1):63–74.
8. Kaminsky DA, Guntupalli KK, Lippmann J, et al. Effect of yoga breathing (pranayama) on exercise tolerance in patients with chronic obstructive pulmonary disease: a randomized, controlled trial. *J Altern Complement Med.* 2017;23(9):696–704.

9. Donesky D. Management of acute breathlessness in the person with chronic refractory breathlessness. *Curr Opin Support Palliat Care*. 2015;9(3):212–216.

10. Mularski RA, Reinke LF, Carrieri-Kohlman V, et al. An official American Thoracic Society workshop report: assessment and palliative management of dyspnea crisis. *Ann Am Thorac Soc*. 2013;10(5):S98–S106.

11. Booth S, Johnson MJ. Improving the quality of life of people with advanced respiratory disease and severe breathlessness. *Breathe (Sheff)*. 2019;15(3):198–215.

5 Treating Episodic Breathlessness

Yvonne Eisenmann and Steffen Simon

A 68-year-old woman with chronic obstructive pulmonary disease (COPD) was hospitalized after being taken to the emergency department with acute respiratory distress. It was the third time in 8 weeks that her husband had called the ambulance when the patient suddenly had severe breathlessness. When she arrived at the emergency department she no longer had breathlessness but gave a vivid description of the symptom and her fear during the episode, including panic, feelings of suffocation, and fear of death. Years ago she had been diagnosed with COPD, and in the past year her respiratory physician had classified it as grade III. Disease-modifying therapy has been optimized and her parameters are stable; her oxygen saturation at check-ups, at admission, and during her hospital stay was in the normal range. Her husband supports her continuously at the hospital and approaches the healthcare professional to ask about therapy and how to prepare for discharge.

What do I do now?

everal short-term and long-term actions should be considered for this woman with a chronic and life-limiting disease. In general, breathlessness is common among patients with advanced malignant and nonmalignant diseases[1] and the prevalence and intensity of breathlessness increase at the end of life.[2] If breathlessness persists despite optimal treatment of the underlying disease and causes disability, it is termed *chronic breathlessness syndrome*.[3] Chronic breathlessness can occur continuously or episodically as a common symptom in palliative care patients.[4] Episodic breathlessness was defined by an international consensus as "characterized by a severe worsening of breathlessness intensity or unpleasantness beyond usual fluctuations in the patient's perception. Episodes are time-limited (seconds to hours) and occur intermittently, with or without underlying continuous breathlessness. Episodes may be predictable or unpredictable, depending on whether any trigger(s) can be identified."[5] The American Thoracic Society likewise defines dyspnea crisis as "severe breathing discomfort that . . . overwhelms the patient and caregiver ability to achieve symptom relief."[6]

Episodic breathlessness involves a complex mechanism of physiological, psychological, social, and environmental factors. Possible sources of the sensation of breathlessness have been discussed,[7] but to date the exact neurophysiological mechanism of breathlessness and the ways that some pharmacological interventions work remain unknown.[8] Chronic breathlessness despite optimal treatment of the underlying disease indicates the need for symptomatic treatment.[3] Management of episodic breathlessness focuses both on the acute clinical situation during the episode of breathlessness and also on long-term interventions (e.g., reducing the number of episodes or improving the patient's ability to cope with episodes).

For patients and family caregivers, episodic breathlessness is a very frightening and burdensome experience with feelings of helplessness. To date, we have some knowledge about the characteristics of breathlessness episodes that can help to support the patient and cope with caring for a breathless patient. Most episodes of breathlessness are short, with a median of 7 minutes for patients with COPD and 5 minutes for patients with cancer; around 9 out of 10 breathlessness episodes last less than 20 minutes. The frequency of episodes differs, but half of the patients experience episodes one to three times a day.[9]

The most common triggers of episodic breathlessness are physical exertion when going up stairs, getting dressed, or speaking.[10] Environmental factors such as warm or cold temperature, high humidity and fog, and exacerbation or acute infections with a fever or a cold can also trigger episodes.[11] Even for episodes initially ranked as unexpected, triggers could usually be identified.[12] Emotions such as anger, trouble, fear, and also great enjoyment or time pressure may develop into episodes of breathlessness despite the absence of physical parameters.[10,11]

Symptoms of depression are common among patients with breathlessness. Anxiety or panic needs clinical attention as it often appears along with breathlessness as either a trigger for breathlessness or as the result of experiencing breathlessness. Experiencing breathlessness and anxiety may develop into a vicious cycle and may reinforce each other. The sensation of breathlessness can lead to feelings of fear and anxiety associated with former experiences of breathlessness, resulting in an increased respiratory rate and muscle tension, which worsens breathlessness.[11,13]

ASSESSMENT

Breathlessness is a subjective symptom and thus can be perceived only by the person experiencing it. Proper assessment is crucial for evaluation and treatment, and self-report of the characteristics of breathlessness episodes is the gold standard.[7]

Reversible causes for which treatment is available (e.g., infections, pleural effusion or embolism) need to be treated. Initial and ongoing assessment during and after treatment enables evaluation of the effectiveness of interventions and ideally involves family caregivers.[11] The characteristics of episodes (e.g., frequency, duration, and intensity) can be determined using a numeric rating scale from 0 (no breathlessness) to 10 (worst breathlessness). Although difficult at first glance, it is often possible to identify triggers for episodic breathlessness. It may help to provide the patient with examples of triggers or to ask the patient to describe the most recent or a typical episode. The patient can provide details on strategies already successfully adopted to relieve symptoms. Attention should be paid to accompanying symptoms such as depression, anxiety, or panic.

TREATMENT

There are several pharmacological and especially nonpharmacological treatment options for episodic breathlessness. Most episodes of breathlessness are over by the time pharmacological options can take effect (e.g., 20 minutes for opioids). Therefore, nonpharmacological interventions are first-line treatments.[9]

The Breathing, Thinking, Functioning (BTF) clinical model[11,13] (Figure 5.1) describes the vicious cycles that worsen breathlessness. The Breathing cycle refers to the pathophysiology of insufficient breathing. The Thinking cycle describes the emotional domain, with increased anxiety and awareness increasing the sensation of breathlessness and resulting into panic. The Functioning cycle specifies deconditioning as a result of reduced activity; muscle deconditioning aggravates breathlessness. The model correspondingly implies strategies to manage breathlessness.

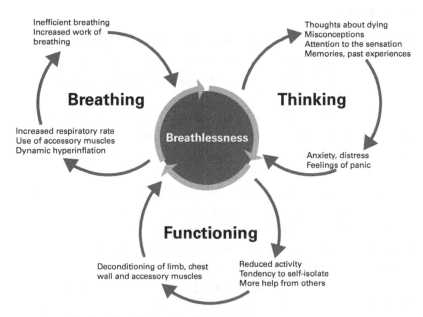

FIGURE 5.1. The Breathing, Thinking, Functioning Model

During an Episode of Breathlessness

During the entire episode of breathlessness, it is essential to stay with patients and calm them down. During episodes breathing is mostly inefficient, as patients breathe quickly and without appropriate tidal volume. Breathing techniques can help patients to reduce their breathing frequency and to enhance deep inspiration for efficient breathing. If possible, the patient should be encouraged during the episode to use pursed-lip breathing or to breathe out longer—for example, while watching the caregiver demonstrating it. Breathing techniques can be taught best in advance when the patient is not breathless. The patient should be encouraged to practice breathing control to prolong expiration and slow down the frequency of breathing. Putting their hands on their belly to feel movement when breathing may help patients to breathe in deeply and to use their respiratory muscles (mainly the diaphragm) instead of moving their upper chest and shoulders.[11]

Using a wet cloth or water spray on the face may reduce breathlessness by providing a sensation of fresh air. Holding a small portable handheld fan in front of the nose, mouth, and cheeks is an easy way to provide fresh air.[14,15] The handheld fan is easy to use and widely available. Also, opening windows or doors to provide a cool breeze may be beneficial. Hypotheses on the potential mechanism of this intervention suggest that receptors of the nasal mucosa and airway induce a decrease in the central respiratory drive, or there may be a placebo effect.[16,17]

Body positioning can help the patient to breathe more effectively.[18] The patient might need help to get into a supportive position, but some patients intuitively adopt a position that helps them breathe more easily. When sitting, they lean forward and rest their arms on their legs or use any furniture to get into a forward-leaning position. It is also possible to help the patient to get into an upright position with arms supported at the side by pillows or an armchair. Again, it is advantageous to teach breathing techniques and beneficial body positions when the patient is not breathless. Health professionals can correct techniques and answer the patient's questions directly.

Preventing Episodic Breathlessness

Patients and caregivers should be taught about breathlessness according to the BTF clinical model, the course of the underlying disease and the symptoms, reasons for being breathless, and strategies to reduce and manage episodes of breathlessness. Written material or web-based tools (YouTube videos) can support knowledge transfer. Letting patients know about the average length of breathlessness episodes and emphasizing that it is only a temporary condition may help them overcome the episode.

Physical exertion, the most common trigger, can be addressed by using pacing strategies. Patients may reduce the intensity or number of their daily activities. They can list their most important activities or duties and consider how they might pace themselves without triggering a breathlessness episode. Mobility aids such as a walking chair that can allow patients to sit for a short rest may help them to pace their activities. Daily activities may be spread out over the day or prioritized starting with the most important one, allowing enough time for recovery. Although being in motion may be strenuous and patients often avoid exercising so as not to trigger an episode of breathlessness, it is important for them to remain active. Exercising helps to maintain bodily fitness because inactivity leads to deconditioning and even more breathlessness when being active.

Cognitive Strategies

Cognitive strategies such as relaxation or distraction techniques can be practiced first in a calm situation before using them during a breathlessness episode. There are several distraction options to take the patient's attention away from breathlessness, such as listening to music, watching television, and reciting a poem or a mantra, and patients should be encouraged to choose their own preferred way. Cognitive-behavioral therapy can address maladaptive thoughts and, in combination with relaxation or diaphragmatic breathing techniques, can help to manage anxiety.[19]

An emergency plan can be helpful for better coping. This plan should be developed together with the patient and family caregiver to increase the feeling of safety and to reduce fear of episodes. This plan may include strategies such as breathing and relaxation techniques, positioning, use of a handheld fan, or any strategies of the patient's choice, including medication when indicated, as well as having a number to call when self-management strategies fail.

Pharmacological Options

Opioids play an important role in the management of chronic breathlessness and are the only drug group with supporting evidence for effective symptom relief.[20,21] For prolonged episodes of breathlessness (duration of 15 minutes and more), opioids can be an option to reduce the burden of breathlessness episodes by taking into account the time of onset and the duration of action. Transmucosal applications of fentanyl are worth a trial and might have some benefit (always being careful with side effects to balance benefit and burden).[22–25]

There is no evidence for the use of benzodiazepines to relieve breathlessness intensity.[22] However, if the patient suffers from anxiety related to breathlessness, it is a therapeutic option to treat the symptom of anxiety and to help the patient better cope with breathlessness and related anxiety.

KEY POINTS TO REMEMBER

- Nonpharmacological interventions are the first-line treatment and support the patient's self-management.
- Stay with the patient during the episode of breathlessness and encourage the patient to use breathing techniques and to take up positions to ease breathing. Keep your own breath calm and encourage the patient to adopt your breathing rhythm.
- Help the patient to cool the face (area of nose, mouth, cheeks) with a handheld fan, open window, or cool water spray.
- Because breathlessness often goes along with anxiety, techniques of relaxation and distraction may reduce anxiety and panic and avoid a vicious circle of breathlessness and panic.
- Educate the patient and family about the duration of breathlessness episodes, triggers, and management strategies.

Further Reading
Booth S, Burkin J, Moffat C, Spathis A, eds. *Managing Breathlessness in Clinical Practice.* Springer; 2014.
Chin C, Booth S. Managing breathlessness: a palliative care approach. *Postgrad Med J.* 2016;92(1089):393–400.

Farquhar M, Penfold C, Benson J, et al. Six key topics informal carers of patients with breathlessness in advanced disease want to learn about and why: MRC phase I study to inform an educational intervention. *PloS One*. 2017;12(5):e0177081.

Simon ST, Weingartner V, Higginson IJ, et al. "I can breathe again!" Patients' self-management strategies for episodic breathlessness in advanced disease, derived from qualitative interviews. *J Pain Symptom Manage*. 2016;52(2):228–234.

Simon ST, Weingärtner V, Higginson IJ, Voltz R, Bausewein C. Definition, categorization, and terminology of episodic breathlessness: consensus by an international Delphi survey. *J Pain Symptom Manage*. 2014;47(5):828–838.

Spathis A, Booth S, Moffat C, et al. The Breathing, Thinking, Functioning clinical model: a proposal to facilitate evidence-based breathlessness management in chronic respiratory disease. *NPJ Prim Care Respir Med*. 2017;27(1):27.

Weingärtner V, Scheve C, Gerdes V, et al. Characteristics of episodic breathlessness as reported by patients with advanced chronic obstructive pulmonary disease and lung cancer: results of a descriptive cohort study. *Palliat Med*. 2015;29(5):420–428.

References

1. Moens K, Higginson IJ, Harding R. Are there differences in the prevalence of palliative care-related problems in people living with advanced cancer and eight non-cancer conditions? A systematic review. *J Pain Symptom Manage*. 2014;48(4):660–677.

2. Currow DC, Smith J, Davidson PM, Newton PJ, Agar MR, Abernethy AP. Do the trajectories of dyspnea differ in prevalence and intensity by diagnosis at the end of life? A consecutive cohort study. *J Pain Symptom Manage*. 2010;39(4):680–690.

3. Johnson MJ, Yorke J, Hansen-Flaschen J, et al. Towards an expert consensus to delineate a clinical syndrome of chronic breathlessness. *Eur Respir J*. 2017;49(5): 1602277.

4. Simon ST, Higginson IJ, Benalia H, et al. Episodic and continuous breathlessness: a new categorization of breathlessness. *J Pain Symptom Manage*. 2013;45(6):1019–1029.

5. Simon ST, Weingärtner V, Higginson IJ, Voltz R, Bausewein C. Definition, categorization, and terminology of episodic breathlessness: consensus by an international Delphi survey. *J Pain Symptom Manage*. 2014;47(5):828–838.

6. Mularski RA, Reinke LF, Carrieri-Kohlman V, et al. An official American Thoracic Society workshop report: assessment and palliative management of dyspnea crisis. *Ann Am Thorac Soc*. 2013;10(5):S98–S106.

7. Parshall MB, Schwartzstein RM, Adams L, et al. An official American Thoracic Society statement: update on the mechanisms, assessment, and management of dyspnea. *Am J Respir Crit Care Med*. 2012;185(4):435–52.

8. Currow DC, Abernethy AP, Allcroft P, et al. The need to research refractory breathlessness. *Eur Respir J*. 2016;47(1):342–343.

9. Weingärtner V, Scheve C, Gerdes V, et al. Characteristics of episodic breathlessness as reported by patients with advanced chronic obstructive pulmonary disease and lung cancer: results of a descriptive cohort study. *Palliat Med*. 2015;29(5):420–428.

10. Simon ST, Bausewein C, Schildmann E, et al. Episodic breathlessness in patients with advanced disease: a systematic review. *J Pain Symptom Manage*. 2013;45(3):561–578.

11. Booth S, Burkin J, Moffat C, Spathis A, eds. *Managing Breathlessness in Clinical Practice*. Springer; 2014.

12. Linde P, Hanke G, Voltz R, Simon ST. Unpredictable episodic breathlessness in patients with advanced chronic obstructive pulmonary disease and lung cancer: a qualitative study. *Support Care Cancer*. 2018;26(4):1097–104.

13. Spathis A, Booth S, Moffat C, et al. The Breathing, Thinking, Functioning clinical model: a proposal to facilitate evidence-based breathlessness management in chronic respiratory disease. *NPJ Prim Care Respir Med*. 2017;27(1):27.

14. Qian MYY, Politis J, Thompson M, et al. Individualized breathlessness interventions may improve outcomes in patients with advanced COPD. *Respirology (Carlton, Vic)*. 2018;23(12):1146–51.

15. Luckett T, Phillips J, Johnson MJ, et al. Contributions of a hand-held fan to self-management of chronic breathlessness. *Eur Respir J*. 2017;50(2):1700262.

16. Liss HP, Grant BJ. The effect of nasal flow on breathlessness in patients with chronic obstructive pulmonary disease. *Am Rev Respir Dis*. 1988;137(6):1285–1288.

17. Swan F, Booth S. The role of airflow for the relief of chronic refractory breathlessness. *Curr Opin Support Palliat Care*. 2015;9(3):206–211.

18. Chin C, Booth S. Managing breathlessness: a palliative care approach. *Postgrad Med J*. 2016;92(1089):393–400.

19. Greer JA, MacDonald JJ, Vaughn J, et al. Pilot study of a brief behavioral intervention for dyspnea in patients with advanced lung cancer. *J Pain Symptom Manage*. 2015;50(6):854–860.

20. Barnes H, McDonald J, Smallwood N, Manser R. Opioids for the palliation of refractory breathlessness in adults with advanced disease and terminal illness. *Cochrane Database Syst Rev*. 2016;3(3):CD011008.

21. Ekstrom M, Nilsson F, Abernethy AA, Currow DC. Effects of opioids on breathlessness and exercise capacity in chronic obstructive pulmonary disease: a systematic review. *Ann Am Thorac Soc*. 2015;12(7):1079–1092.

22. Simon ST, Kloke M, Alt-Epping B, et al. EffenDys-fentanyl buccal tablet for the relief of episodic breathlessness in patients with advanced cancer: a multicenter, open-label, randomized, morphine-controlled, crossover, phase II trial. *J Pain Symptom Manage*. 2016;52(5):617–625.

23. Hui D, Kilgore K, Frisbee-Hume S, et al. Effect of prophylactic fentanyl buccal tablet on episodic exertional dyspnea: a pilot double-blind randomized controlled trial. *J Pain Symptom Manage*. 2017;54(6):798–805.
24. Hui D, Kilgore K, Park M, Williams J, Liu D, Bruera E. Impact of prophylactic fentanyl pectin nasal spray on exercise-induced episodic dyspnea in cancer patients: a double-blind, randomized controlled trial. *J Pain Symptom Manage*. 2016;52(4):459–468.
25. Hui D, Xu A, Frisbee-Hume S, et al. Effects of prophylactic subcutaneous fentanyl on exercise-induced breakthrough dyspnea in cancer patients: a preliminary double-blind, randomized, controlled trial. *J Pain Symptom Manage*. 2014;47(2):209–217.

6   Reducing Episodic Dyspnea in Heart Failure

Beth B. Fahlberg and Ann S. Laramee

A 66-year-old man presents to the emergency department with dyspnea for the past 3 days. His 25-year cardiac history includes a stent for myocardial infarction a year ago, heart failure (HF), an implantable cardioverter defibrillator (ICD), and cardiorenal syndrome. He also has chronic obstructive pulmonary disease (COPD). This dyspnea episode began 3 days ago, exacerbated by exertion and lying flat in bed, prompting him to sleep in a recliner. Seeking relief, he called his pulmonologist's office but was told it sounded like his heart and to call cardiology. The cardiology nurse said it was probably a lung problem given his recent exacerbation and no weight gain, and to call the pulmonologist. Frustrated at being turfed between specialists and not getting help, he called 911. He didn't know whether his dyspnea was due to his heart or his lungs; he just knew he couldn't breathe.

What do I do now?

This is a common situation: A patient presents with dyspnea, but the cause is not straightforward. Is the dyspnea due to fluid overload from his HF, another COPD exacerbation, pneumonia, or a longer-term consequence of his COVID-19? Or, is this episode of dyspnea multifactorial, a combination of all these problems? Even more challenging, how can we prevent recurrent episodes of dyspnea and recurrent hospitalization moving forward in this high-risk patient?

ASSESSMENT

A targeted assessment of the patient's cardiopulmonary status is an important first step in determining the correct course of action. Assessment should first focus on the patient's clinical stability and need for emergent or urgent intervention. Next, look for signs and symptoms specific to the suspected causes of his dyspnea. Diagnosis of HF requires both symptoms and corresponding clinical signs. To determine if the patient's dyspnea is caused by HF-related fluid overload, you should look for orthopnea, jugular vein distention (JVD), bibasilar crackles, ascites, peripheral edema, and weight gain, as described next.

Orthopnea

This patient reports dyspnea when lying down (orthopnea) and is sleeping in a recliner. Orthopnea is strongly suggestive of HF-related pulmonary congestion due to fluid overload.[1] Patients should be asked if they have started propping up with pillows in bed, sleeping in a recliner, or even sitting up to sleep or breathe more easily. Orthopnea may be observed clinically when the person has dyspnea in a supine position that resolves with elevating the head of bed or exam table.[2]

JVD

This clinical sign is also strongly suggestive of HF-related fluid overload,[1] as the jugular veins are an outward sign of the pressure inside the heart. Proper positioning and pressure on the upper right abdomen can aid in detecting subtle changes in JVD, but when the patient is sitting up comfortably and their jugular vein is distended up to their jawline, you know they have pulmonary congestion and fluid overload. Clinicians working with HF patients should become comfortable with assessment for JVD.

Bibasilar Crackles

Lung sounds in fluid overload often demonstrate bibasilar crackles, moving up the lung fields bilaterally with increasing severity. However, the absence of crackles does not rule out pulmonary congestion as lymphatic drainage can increase to compensate for chronic pulmonary congestion.[2]

Ascites

Fluid retention in HF may be focused in the abdomen, with or without peripheral edema. Look for abdominal distention and fluid wave on your examination.[2] Ask the patient whether their pants have been tight, they have felt bloated, or they had a poor appetite or early satiety.

Peripheral Edema

While not specific to HF, new or worsening peripheral edema is often suggestive of fluid overload. HF-related edema is bilateral, pitting, and dependent, starting in the feet and ankles and moving up the legs with additional fluid retention, or settling in the sacrum of bed-bound patients.[2]

Weight Gain

Increasing weight often accompanies worsening fluid retention. However, weight gain has poor specificity as a clinical sign of fluid overload. This is common in advanced heart failure, when gradual fluid retention can be disguised by the weight loss that occurs toward the end of life with the development of frailty and cardiac cachexia.[2]

ETIOLOGY

If HF is identified as the cause of symptoms, try to determine the cause of the exacerbation to better target therapies. Common cardiac etiologies of an episode of worsening dyspnea in HF include ischemia or new myocardial infarction, hypertension, arrhythmias, atrial fibrillation, not being on guideline-directed medical therapies (GDMTs), high dietary sodium intake, medication nonadherence, and disease progression. However, if the cause of dyspnea is still not clear, ordering a brain natriuretic peptide (BNP) level and chest x-ray can help.

BNP

Dyspnea may have several different causes, so identification of increased natriuretic peptide levels (BNP or N-terminal-prohormone BNP [NT-proBNP]) is useful in confirming HF as the primary cause for the patient's dyspnea.[3] Natriuretic peptide levels increase with worsening fluid overload. An increase from the patient's baseline can distinguish between cardiac and respiratory dyspnea or other noncardiac etiologies. The BNP level associated with symptomatic fluid overload is highly individualized; therefore, results should be compared with previous findings and correlated with the patient's symptoms and exam findings.[2]

Chest X-Ray

Chest x-ray findings in pulmonary congestion due to HF may show pleural effusions, cardiomegaly, upper lobe pulmonary venous congestion, and pulmonary or interstitial edema. In contrast, x-ray findings associated with pneumonia include airspace opacity, lobar consolidation, or interstitial opacities. With COPD, enlarged lungs, air pockets (bullae), or a flattened diaphragm may be found on chest x-ray.

OTHER DIAGNOSTICS

Ejection Fraction

Determining a patient's ejection fraction (EF) will help guide the use of evidence-based HF therapies, particularly in low-EF heart failure. A normal EF is usually between 50% and 70%. In HF, EF is classified as either reduced (<40%), borderline (41–49%), or preserved (>50%).[1] EF is typically determined using echocardiogram (ECHO). Look for the most recent ECHO reports or cardiology progress notes to find this in the electronic medical record. A new ECHO can be done to assess for changes in EF or valve function that may be responsible for the patient's current symptoms, particularly if they have been stable until this episode.

Renal Function and Potassium

Close monitoring of renal function, electrolytes, and fluid status is essential when assessing and treating fluid overload as all are interrelated and can be impacted by worsening cardiac function and diuretic treatments.[1,4]

Interrogation of Cardiac Electrical Device

Interrogation of a cardiac device such as an ICD or pacemaker can help identify other factors contributing to HF exacerbation. Device data can be used to identify the burden of atrial fibrillation, the average heart rate, or arrhythmias that may be contributing to HF symptoms. Ask the patient for their device wallet card, which has information about their device, and contact a nurse in electrophysiology or cardiology for assistance with device interrogation.

TREATMENT

Diuresis

Diuresis is the cornerstone of treatment for dyspnea associated with pulmonary congestion in HF (Box 6.1). Daily doses of oral loop diuretics are the key to managing fluid overload and preventing dyspnea in HF. While furosemide is the most common loop diuretic used, bumetanide and torsemide, which have a better bioavailability and duration of action, may be more effective in patients who develop diuretic resistance. Acute episodes of dyspnea usually require intravenous diuretics.

The right dose of diuretic is often specific to the individual's diuretic threshold, which is the dose that measurably increases the urine output within 2 hours. A minimal diuretic response usually requires doubling the dose, while post-dose sodium retention requires twice-a-day dosing.

Careful and close monitoring of fluid status is essential to avoid adverse effects of overdiuresis such as symptomatic orthostatic hypotension, which can cause falls. Monitoring should include assessing for changes in physical exam findings of fluid overload, checking daily weights, watching for a return to the patient's baseline dry weight, and symptom improvement. A worsening creatinine concentration is common with diuresis and is usually transient, so if fluid overload persists, ongoing diuresis will be necessary. Once euvolemia is obtained, a maintenance diuretic dose or an as-needed (prn) dose of oral diuretic will need to be determined based on ongoing assessments.

Cardiorenal syndrome and diuretic resistance are common in advanced HF. Strategies to treat dyspnea related to fluid overload in these patients can include using higher doses of oral diuretics, intermittent intravenous diuretics, or prn oral metolazone.[4] Close monitoring of renal function, potassium, and fluid status is essential as metolazone is highly potent and can quickly lead to symptomatic dehydration and hypokalemia associated with arrhythmias, ICD discharges, or even sudden cardiac death.

GDMTs

GDMTs are the cornerstone of HF treatment and include procedures, surgeries, devices, and medications. GDMTs are used to modify the underlying structural or functional heart problem(s) identified as the probable cause of the patient's HF symptoms.[1] Look at the big picture to determine which HF therapies to recommend for the individual patient. This includes identifying the patient's stage of HF, their status on the disease trajectory, and their overall prognosis, considering signs of frailty and their comorbidities.[2]

Dietary Sodium Restriction

Sodium restriction is commonly recommended to patients with HF to prevent fluid overload, though scientific evidence to support this practice is lacking.[1] Current guidelines state that "clinicians should consider some degree of sodium restriction (e.g., <3 g) in patients with stage C and D HF for symptom improvement."[1]

Treat Comorbid Conditions

For patients with advanced HF, optimizing the treatment of comorbid conditions usually improves their HF symptoms, including dyspnea.[5]

Additional Pharmacological Strategies

When patients have refractory dyspnea despite optimized management of HF medications, fluid status, and other comorbid conditions, consider inotropic infusion therapy and/or symptom relief with opioids or benzodiazepines,[6] consistent with their goals of care.[2,7]

Additional Nonpharmacological Strategies

Nonpharmacological strategies can be essential in effectively managing HF-related dyspnea. Positioning for comfortable breathing is often indispensable (e.g., elevating the head and torso in bed, in a recliner, or in a hospital bed at home). Other strategies for dyspnea management include home oxygen for hypoxia, using a fan to circulate air, relaxation techniques, pursed-lip breathing, providing a calm, peaceful atmosphere, pulmonary rehabilitation, and integrative therapies.[2]

PREVENTING DYSPNEA RECURRENCE

Evidence-based strategies to prevent HF exacerbations include optimizing GDMTs, follow-up visits within a week of HF discharge, and patient and family education to monitor, recognize, and manage symptoms.[8] In addition, the following strategies can also be effective in preventing recurrent dyspnea and should be individualized to the patient and their symptoms, treatment preferences, and resources.[2]

Symptom and Weight Home Monitoring

A key to preventing recurrent dyspnea in HF is home monitoring for early recognition and treatment of fluid overload. This includes daily monitoring for weight gain and worsening HF symptoms such as dyspnea, orthopnea, and edema. Home monitoring may be done short-term after hospitalization or long-term in patients with advanced HF and recurrent exacerbations. Many monitoring options are available, and most healthcare organizations, insurance companies, and HMOs will either have their own HF program or contract with an HF monitoring service, usually run by nurses certified in HF care.

Symptom Management Plans

A patient-focused symptom management plan developed in conjunction with the patient and their caregiver is also essential to effective symptom management in HF-related episodic dyspnea. This plan includes what they should do for worsening symptoms, increasing weight, or episodes of distressing dyspnea. Recommended strategies may include prn diuretic doses, positioning, anxiety control, and other nonpharmacological and pharmacological interventions. The symptom management plan should also include one number to call where they can get help for whatever is going on in order to prevent the type of situation seen in our case, where the patient was sent from one specialist to another without help. The plan should be individualized and should include both evidence-based interventions appropriate for the patient and their symptoms and other strategies that work for the patient. An effective plan should promote early intervention for fluid overload, increase the patient's and caregiver's control over the symptoms, decrease their anxiety, and hopefully prevent unnecessary emergency visits and 911 calls.

Advance Care Planning

In HF, as in other conditions, planning for the future should be done in the context of a patient's overall values, wishes, and goals of care to ensure appropriate, concordant care.[7] This has been shown to improve quality of life, patient satisfaction with end-of-life care, and end-of-life communication.[7,9] Issues pertinent in HF include the following:

Would invasive diagnostic tests, procedures, or surgery be acceptable?
What about mechanical ventilation?
Would they consider advanced HF therapies or long-term dialysis?

Discussion about the option of deactivating ICD defibrillation capabilities should be included in any discussion about cardiopulmonary resuscitation (CPR) preferences,[7] and ICD deactivation should be a separate decision from a do-not-resuscitate order.[2]

CONCLUSION

The patient described at the beginning of this chapter was taken by ambulance to the emergency department. His BNP level was 1270, twice his baseline of 580 a year ago. He exhibited significant orthopnea and dyspnea with exertion and reported episodic dyspnea several times per day with any activity. While his weight was stable (256 lbs compared with 257 lbs 3 months ago and 255 lbs a year ago), muscle wasting and frailty were notable, disguising his fluid retention. JVD was prominent, increasing with upper right abdominal pressure. While there was no peripheral edema, his pants were tight. Serum creatinine was increased, 2.5 compared to a 1.9 baseline, and his potassium level was 4.5 (within normal limits). Chest x-ray revealed no signs of pneumonia or COVID-19 changes, ECHO showed his EF had dropped from 35% to 25%, and interrogation of his ICD showed no atrial fibrillation or other clinically significant arrhythmias. He was diagnosed with acute-on-chronic advanced HF. Treatment included diuresis with intravenous furosemide and up-titration of his angiotensin-converting-enzyme (ACE) inhibitor. His symptom management plan included prn furosemide for increased weight. Assessment of his self-care practices revealed strong adherence to his complex medication regimen and dietary sodium restriction, and a self-imposed limit on fluid intake of 2 liters per day. He started home HF monitoring with telehealth support through his Medicare provider, and at follow-up visits reported fewer episodes of symptomatic dyspnea.

- Assessment and diagnostic test findings in HF-related dyspnea include orthopnea, JVD, bibasilar crackles, ascites, peripheral edema, weight gain, elevated BNP levels, and pulmonary congestion on chest x-ray.
- Symptomatic management of dyspnea due to fluid overload in HF requires diuresis, as well as treatment of the underlying etiology, which may include cardiac or noncardiac issues, medication titration, and working with the patient on self-care strategies, including restriction of dietary sodium intake and medication adherence.
- A patient-focused symptom management plan may include prn diuretic doses for increased weight, positioning for comfort, and anxiety reduction approaches to managing dyspnea at home.

References

1. Yancy CW, Jessup M, Bozkurt B, et al. 2013 ACCF/AHA guideline for the management of heart failure: a report of the American College of Cardiology Foundation/American Heart Association Task Force on practice guidelines. *Circulation*. 2013;128(16):e240–e327.

2. Panke JT, Donaho E, Fahlberg BB. *Compendium of Treatment of End-Stage Non-Cancer Diagnoses: Heart Failure* (3rd ed.; Whitehead P, ed.). Kendall/Hunt; 2020.

3. Yancy CW, Jessup M, Bozkurt B, et al. 2017 ACC/AHA/HFSA focused update of the 2013 ACCF/AHA guideline for the management of heart failure: a report of the American College of Cardiology/American Heart Association Task Force on Clinical Practice Guidelines and the Heart Failure Society of America. *Circulation*. 2017;136(6):e137–e161.

4. Felker MG, Ellison DH, Mullens W, Cox ZL, Testani JM. Diuretic therapy for patients with heart failure. *J Am Coll Cardiol*. 2020;75(10):1178–1195.

5. Yancy CW, Januzzi JL Jr, Allen LA, et al. 2017 ACC expert consensus decision pathway for optimization of heart failure treatment: answers to 10 pivotal issues about heart failure with reduced ejection fraction: a report of the American College of Cardiology Task Force on Expert Consensus Decision Pathways. *J Am Coll Cardiol*. 2018;71(2):201–230.

6. Mahler DA, Selecky PA, Harrod CG, et al. American College of Chest Physicians consensus statement on the management of dyspnea in patients with advanced lung or heart disease. *Chest*. 2010;137(3):674–691.

7. Braun LT, Grady KL, Kutner JS, et al. Palliative care and cardiovascular disease and stroke: a policy statement from the American Heart Association/American Stroke Association. *Circulation*. 2016;134(11):e198–e225.

8. Rasmusson K, Flattery M, Baas LS. American Association of Heart Failure Nurses position paper on educating patients with heart failure. *Heart Lung*. 2015;44(2):173–177.

9. Schichtel M, Wee B, Perera R, Onakpoya I, Albury C, Barber S. Clinician-targeted interventions to improve advance care planning in heart failure: a systematic review and meta-analysis. *Heart*. 2019;105(17):1316–1324.

7 Dyspnea in Pediatric Congenital Heart Disease

Jennifer Wright and Jessica L. Spruit

RR is a 12-year-old male with a complex congenital cardiac history. He was born with hypoplastic left heart syndrome (HLHS) variant, leaving him with single ventricle physiology. He underwent staged surgical palliation; however, due to his complex anatomy, he was unable to move beyond the hemi-Fontan palliation surgery. Surgery left him with significant cyanosis at baseline further complicated by severe asthma He was admitted with increased work of breathing, diaphoresis, and lightheadedness in the setting of prolonged arrhythmia with low cardiac output. RR appeared to be in relative respiratory distress; however, he reported this was his baseline and denied discomfort at rest but has increased work of breathing with shortness of breath with activity. He developed new complications secondary to low cardiac output; he is requiring continuous renal replacement therapy for acute kidney failure and increased pulmonary edema. RR is increasingly symptomatic with dyspnea in the setting of organ failure.

What do I do now?

As a clinician approaching this case, one immediate challenge is the recognition of dyspnea. Patients with congenital heart disease often live with dyspnea without distress at baseline, complicating the ability of the patient and clinician to recognize when dyspnea becomes a symptom of distress and to intervene appropriately. Due to the possible presence of underlying dyspnea in the child with cyanotic congenital heart disease, it is essential that the clinician determine whether or not the patient's symptoms deviate from their "healthy" baseline. Even more important, the clinician is charged with the responsibility of determining whether or not the symptoms are perceived by the patient as bothersome or uncomfortable. Often, the palliative care clinician may not be engaged in such cases until very late in the course of disease given this tolerance of baseline dyspnea and narrow margin of respiratory reserve.

When approaching RR's care, it is important to first consider the etiology of his symptoms, confirming the relationship of his congenital heart disease to the dyspnea he is experiencing. It is necessary to determine whether or not his asthma may in fact be the primary etiology of increasing respiratory distress. Asthma as the cause of RR's distress was ruled out as he failed to respond to interventions targeting the pathophysiology of asthma. This should prompt the clinician to proceed with an evaluation of his cardiac status. This evaluation may include laboratory studies, chest x-ray, electrocardiograph, echocardiogram, and cardiac catheterization.

The extent and invasiveness of the evaluation should be guided by the goals of treatment. An initial assessment will likely include laboratory studies, a chest x-ray, electrocardiograph, and echocardiogram. If goals of care are fully comfort-focused, this may be the extent of diagnostic studies performed. Laboratory values will help to identify renal function and acid–base balance. The chest x-ray will be interpreted to identify any pulmonary infiltrates, consolidation, or pleural effusions that may cause dyspnea or evidence of pulmonary vascular congestion. An electrocardiograph will assist in the identification of arrhythmias, such as atrial tachyarrhythmias that are common in patients who underwent Fontan.[1] Echocardiographs are used to evaluate the structure and function of the heart and will assist in assessment of blood flow. Infectious testing to determine if the dyspnea can be attributed to a respiratory infectious illness may be warranted. If RR and his family desire continued medical treatment and may consider further intervention focused on prolonging life, information gained from a cardiac catheterization may be used to guide discussion about whether he is a candidate for additional interventional or surgical palliation. Cardiac catheterization will assist in measurement of pressures and explore the role of vascular volume in the presentation of dyspnea.

In this case, RR was experiencing dyspnea as a result of pulmonary overcirculation due to his complex congenital heart defect. HLHS is a cyanotic defect that can result in pulmonary overcirculation and diminished cardiac output (Figure 7.1). The initial approach to RR's dyspnea will target the underlying pathophysiology and provide interventions for symptom relief. Much of the information available regarding treatment of heart failure and dyspnea in the pediatric population is extrapolated from adult information. There is limited pediatric information available in the literature to guide clinical decision-making for pediatric providers.[2,3] Collaboration with colleagues from pediatric cardiology supports the medical management of pulmonary overcirculation and heart failure in this case.

FLUID MANAGEMENT

Diuretic therapy is an initial intervention to manage the fluid overload and pulmonary overcirculation that RR is experiencing as a consequence of his HLHS defect. Diuresis and natriuresis are achieved through the administration of loop diuretics.[3] The two most commonly used diuretics in pediatric heart failure are furosemide and bumetanide.[3] Thiazide diuretics may also be used in the setting of pediatric heart failure; they are frequently administered in combination with loop diuretics.[3] Chlorothiazide and hydrochlorothiazide are two commonly used thiazide diuretics in pediatric heart failure.[4] In the setting of diuretic resistance, many other agents may be trialed for volume overload, including

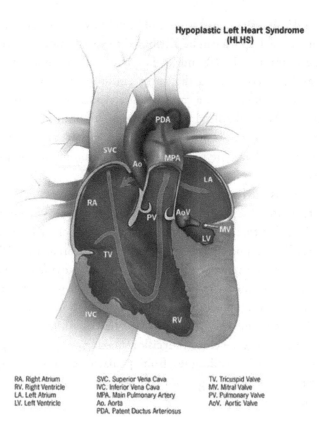

Hypoplastic Left Heart Syndrome
(HLHS)

RA. Right Atrium	SVC. Superior Vena Cava	TV. Tricuspid Valve
RV. Right Ventricle	IVC. Inferior Vena Cava	MV. Mitral Valve
LA. Left Atrium	MPA. Main Pulmonary Artery	PV. Pulmonary Valve
LV. Left Ventricle	Ao. Aorta	AoV. Aortic Valve
	PDA. Patent Ductus Arteriosus	

FIGURE 7.1.   Hypoplastic left heart syndrome

concurrent administration of albumin with loop diuretic therapy, dopamine to improve renal perfusion and urine production, fenoldopam to promote vasodilation of the renal arteries and increase urine output, and nesiritide to promote arterial and venous vasodilation, which modulates the renin–angiotensin–aldosterone system (RAAS) and promotes diuresis and natriuresis.[3] Ultimately, continuous renal replacement therapy was required in RR's case given his acute kidney failure secondary to hypoxemia and hypoperfusion.

AFTERLOAD REDUCTION

Decreasing the systemic vascular resistance in single-ventricle physiology will help reduce the shunting of blood to the pulmonary vasculature and relieve some of the pulmonary vascular congestion that produces dyspnea. First-line pharmacotherapy for afterload reduction in children with heart failure is angiotensin-converting-enzyme (ACE) inhibitors, which work through decreased formation of angiotensin II, blocked formation of the RAAS, and decreased adrenergic activity. ACE inhibitors have been shown to improve symptoms, reduce progression of heart failure, and improve survival in adult trials. Captopril, enalapril, and lisinopril are among the ACE inhibitors used for afterload reduction in pediatric heart failure. The efficacy of angiotensin receptor blockers (ARBs) has also been documented in the adult literature, especially in cases of adults who are not tolerant of ACE inhibitor therapy. Commonly used ARBs include spironolactone and eplerenone. Large pediatric trials of either pharmacological class have not been performed, but they are part of the consensus guidelines.[4]

Beta-receptor antagonist therapy has also demonstrated improvement in symptoms and ejection fraction in pediatric studies. Carvedilol and metoprolol are among the most commonly used beta-blockers in pediatric data. Inotropic agents including dopamine, dobutamine, and milrinone may also be used in the setting of acute decompensation with impaired perfusion. It is important to note that if the perfusion is preserved, even in the setting of congestion, inotropic agents may be harmful and should not be used.[4]

NONPHARMACOLOGICAL INTERVENTIONS FOR DYSPNEA

While evidence supports several nonpharmacological interventions in adults with dyspnea, there is a paucity of pediatric evidence in the literature. Interventions that may be attempted include cooling the room and providing a fan to promote cool airflow to the face of a child or adolescent with dyspnea. Self-regulation techniques such as guided imagery, mindfulness, and deep breathing may relieve the experience of dyspnea, although there is not clear evidence to support these interventions. Smartphone apps are available to support exercises such as this. Many children and adolescents with congenital heart disease use interventions such as this without recognizing that they are palliating dyspnea.[2]

PHARMACOLOGICAL INTERVENTIONS FOR DYSPNEA

In the treatment of dyspnea in adults there is a clear benefit of morphine and fentanyl, which are effective at reducing air hunger and ventilatory response to decreased oxygen and increased carbon dioxide through altered central perception.[2] Opioids may be administered via the oral, intranasal, or intravenous routes. Use of intranasal fentanyl has been supported by small studies in the pediatric population from newborns to adolescents.[5,6] Consideration of patient variables will guide the selection of the preferred opioid and route of administration. As a standard in pain management, opioid therapy is often initiated with short-acting agents, and may be transitioned to longer-acting formulations when symptoms stabilize, as part of maintenance therapy. Evidence does not exist to guide the clinician in initiating a specific formulation or determining doses of opioids for dyspnea relief, but initial doses are often approximately 25–50% of the dose that would be administered to treat pain in opioid-naïve children.[2,7] Patients who have been on opioid therapy for pain will often require an increase in their opioid doses when dyspnea management is required; adult studies report increases by 25% of their breakthrough pain doses[2] or 10–15% of total daily requirements.[8] Opioids commonly used in pediatric dyspnea include morphine and fentanyl.[2,6]

Although not recommended as monotherapy in the absence of opioids, benzodiazepines may also be useful in the relief of anxiety that often accompanies the sensation of breathlessness.[2,7,9] Among the anxiolytics used in pediatric palliative care, midazolam is often administered via intranasal or buccal routes.[2]

PROGRESSIVE NATURE OF HEART FAILURE

Multiple factors complicate the recognition and assessment of dyspnea in pediatric congenital heart disease. Patients often experience a baseline dyspnea throughout their lives and may not recognize progressive symptoms as a result of this underlying tolerance. Additionally, out of necessity, many patients have learned strategies for management of dyspnea without realizing that is what they are achieving. Examples of this include the frequent report of children preferring cool rooms with a fan blowing on them, or mobilizing relaxation techniques for dyspnea that is often perceived solely as "anxiety." This poses a challenge for the clinician caring for a patient with congenital heart disease, as the recognition of symptoms may correlate with significant decline in cardiac function and rapid progression toward the end of life.

KEY POINTS TO REMEMBER

- Dyspnea in pediatric congenital heart disease may be difficult to recognize given the baseline respiratory distress that patients with this history experience.
- Medical management of pulmonary overcirculation may be achieved with diuresis and afterload reduction.
- Dyspnea secondary to congenital heart disease may be managed as dyspnea from other causes is managed; nonpharmacological and pharmacological agents may be used, increasing in aggressiveness as goals of care transition.
- Pediatric patients experiencing dyspnea in the setting of congenital heart disease may present late in their disease process, requiring clinicians to recognize and relieve their distress and facilitate values-guided shared decision-making promptly.

Further Reading
Mazwi ML, Henner N, Kirsch R. The role of palliative care in critical congenital heart disease. *Semin Perinatol.* 2017;41:128–132.

References
1. Guccione P, Iorio FS, Rebonato M, et al. Profiles of heart failure in adolescents and young adults with congenital heart disease. *Prog Pediatr Cardiol.* 2018;51:37–45.
2. Craig F, Henderson EM, Bluebond-Langner M. Management of respiratory symptoms in paediatric palliative care. *Curr Opin Support Palliat Care.* 2015;9(3):217–226.
3. McCammond AN, Axelrod DM, Bailly DK, Ramsey EZ, Costello JM. Pediatric cardiac intensive care society 2014 consensus statement: pharmacotherapies

in cardiac critical care fluid management. *Pediatr Crit Care Med.* 2016;17(supp 3):S35–S48.

4. Rossano JW, Cabrera AG, Jefferies JL, Naim MY, Humlicek T. Pediatric cardiac intensive care society 2014 consensus statement: pharmacotherapies in cardiac critical care chronic heart failure. *Pediatr Crit Care Med.* 2016;17(supp 3):S20–S34.

5. Harlos MS, Stenekes S, Lambert D, Hohl C, Chochinov HM. Intranasal fentanyl in the palliative care of newborns and infants. *J Pain Symptom Manage.* 2013;46(2):265–274.

6. Pieper L, Wager J, Zernikow B. Intranasal fentanyl for respiratory distress in children and adolescents with life-limiting conditions. *BMC Palliat Care.* 2018;17:106–113.

7. Robinson WM. Palliation of dyspnea in pediatrics. *Chronic Respir Dis.* 2012;9(4):251–256.

8. Stewart D, McPherson ML. Symptom management challenges in heart failure: pharmacotherapy considerations. *Heart Fail Rev.* 2017;22(5):525–534.

9. Pieper L, Zernikow B, Drake R, Frosch M, Printz M, Wagner J. Dyspnea in children with life-threatening and life-limiting complex chronic conditions. *J Palliat Med.* 2018;21(4):552–564.

8 Treating Chronic Dyspnea in Patients with Lung Cancer

Elizabeth A. Higgins, Susan Ezemenari, and Julia Arana West

A 63-year-old male on home oxygen presents to the hospital complaining of shortness of breath. He has a history of metastatic poorly differentiated squamous cell carcinoma of the lung which was diagnosed 3 months prior to this visit. He has received two cycles of pembrolizumab and tolerated it well. He has also received palliative radiation therapy to some painful bony metastases in his pelvis and lumbar spine. The patient has a history of chronic obstructive pulmonary disease (COPD), hypertension, and hyperlipidemia. His blood pressure is 145/54 (no pulsus paradoxus); his pulse is 93 and his oxygen saturation is 100% on 2 L via nasal cannula. Examination is notable for decreased breath sounds at both bases and clubbing of the fingers. Innumerable pulmonary nodules and a right middle lobe mass are present and largely unchanged from his last CT.

What do I do now?

Dyspnea is the subjective experience of difficulty breathing and includes the physical and emotional distress that may accompany this feeling. Descriptors that are often used interchangeably are shortness of breath or air hunger; dyspnea is multifactorial in etiology, impact, and intervention. Its prevalence is up to 78% in cancer patients and 56% in non-cancer patients. Dyspnea can greatly impact quality of life as it diminishes functional status, social activities, and the will to live. Interestingly, terminal sedation is prompted three times more by dyspnea than by pain.

The subjective experience of dyspnea is mediated by both neural and sensory input. Mechanoreceptors of the lung parenchyma, chest wall, diaphragm, and airway, plus chemoreceptors of the medulla and the carotid and aortic bodies provide input to the sensory cortex and medulla. The medulla in turn stimulates respiratory muscles and provides feedback to the sensory cortex. Imaging studies suggest that the sensation of dyspnea is processed cortically in the anterior insula and amygdala.

While there are certain signs that often accompany dyspnea (e.g., tachypnea, accessory muscle use, paradoxical breathing. and nasal flaring), in the palliative setting the patient report of dyspnea is considered the most reliable measurement for the presence and severity of this symptom. In other words, normal respiratory rate or normal oxygen saturation does not preclude the presence of dyspnea. Conversely, tachypnea and/or hypoxemia may not signify dyspnea for the patient with chronic disease such as COPD.

Dyspnea is a common complaint in both the emergency/acute care and primary care settings. As a symptom it is associated with myriad chronic, acute-on-chronic, and acute/reversible pathologies. It is important to differentiate between these etiologies to direct treatment (with or without "curative intent") and symptom management. Some potentially reversible causes of dyspnea may be pain, pleural effusion, pneumonia, and abdominal ascites.

Regardless of its origin, dyspnea is a complex subjective experience that is physical and psychological. Dyspnea in cancer patients is even more complex as there is often more than one factor contributing to the symptom. Primary or metastatic involvement of the lung or pleura with cancer is a common etiology. Many patients with lung cancer have a history of smoking and may have dyspnea from COPD. Respiratory muscle weakness has been associated with the presence of dyspnea, but the severity of abnormal spirometry has not been shown to predict the severity of dyspnea.

Screening for dyspnea using a validated tool such as the Edmond Symptom Assessment scale (ESAS) is a first step in recognizing the presence of dyspnea. The ESAS is designed to assist in the assessment of nine symptoms common in cancer patients. The severity at the time of the assessment of each symptom is rated from 0 to 10 on a numeric scale, with 0 meaning that the symptom is absent and 10 that it is the worst possible severity. The ESAS provides a clinical profile of symptom severity over time and can be administered in the palliative outpatient clinic, in palliative home care, and in the inpatient consult setting.

In the case above, the likely cause of dyspnea is progression of lung cancer. Although the patient's chest CT scan showed innumerable pulmonary nodules and a right middle lobe mass that is largely unchanged from previous imaging, his advanced disease (no response after two cycles of immunotherapy) and his functional decline suggest that his disease has progressed. Pembrolizumab may be associated with dyspnea in 10–23% of patients (mostly from immune-mediated pneumonitis), but this patient's CT showed no interstitial edema. Also, on physical exam, he had decreased breath sounds on both lung bases, which may suggest pulmonary effusion or edema, but this should have been seen on chest CT if it were present. The mechanism of dyspnea in lung cancer includes extrinsic or intraluminal airway obstruction, obstructive pneumonitis or atelectasis, lymphangitis, tumor spread, tumor emboli, pneumothorax, pleural effusion, or pericardial effusion with tamponade. The differential diagnosis of dyspnea includes the advancement of lung cancer, pneumonia, superior vena cava syndrome, pulmonary embolism, malignant pleural effusion, pneumothorax, or radiation pneumonitis. The patient's symptoms may also be caused by a COPD exacerbation or treatment-related pneumonitis from chest radiation, immunotherapy, and/or chemotherapy. He may also have pulmonary edema due to heart failure, a pericardial effusion, an acid–base disturbance, anemia, pain or anxiety.

The workup of this patient should include obtaining a CBC to check for anemia, a complete metabolic profile to look for metabolic abnormalities, a B-type natriuretic peptide to look for heart failure, and possibly an arterial blood gas to check for acid–base disorders. Of course one should obtain a chest radiograph to look for consolidation, interstitial edema, effusions, and a pneumothorax. A CT angiogram of the chest should be considered to exclude pulmonary embolism.

Treatment of reversible causes of dyspnea should include treatment for a COPD exacerbation with bronchodilators, steroids, and noninvasive positive-pressure ventilation (NIPPV). If heart failure is present, then one should treat with diuretics, nitrates, NIPPV, and other disease-modifying therapies. Pulmonary embolism should be treated with anticoagulation if there is no contraindication. A patient who is dyspneic from anemia may feel better after a blood transfusion. Pneumonia would be treated with antibiotics, and a pleural effusion/cardiac tamponade would be treated with decompression. If the patient is anxious, benzodiazepines may be useful. Pain should be treated with opioids, which will also relieve dyspnea.

Nonpharmacological interventions for dyspnea include chest wall vibration, walking aids, and breathing training. People who are short of breath often obtain relief by sitting near an open window or in front of a fan. Patients with dyspnea should avoid smoke and strong odors and may find relief by sitting upright and supporting their upper arms on a table. Pursed-lip breathing also slows the respiratory rate and increases airway pressure and may help patients who have increased dyspnea. Formal muscle relaxation techniques may decrease anxiety and breathlessness, and guided imagery may be a useful adjunctive therapy. Existential concerns that may contribute to breathlessness and anxiety should also be addressed, ideally by a professional chaplain.

The usefulness of oxygen to relieve dyspnea is not clear. In the hypoxic patient with COPD such as in this case, oxygen supplementation may improve survival, pulmonary hemodynamics, exercise capacity, and neuropsychological performance. In the non-hypoxic individual, oxygen does not provide additional benefit compared with room air for the relief of breathlessness. Despite lack of clear evidence of the benefit of oxygen in the terminal patient, some terminally ill patients report a marked improvement in both breathlessness and quality of life with the use of oxygen. Oxygen may be useful when patients are experiencing distress or are hypoxemic, but it should not be initiated if the patient is feeling comfortable and is near death.

Systemic opioids are the first-line treatment of dyspnea associated with advanced lung cancer. Even a single bolus dose of morphine can significantly improve dyspnea. The mechanism of action of opioids may include decreasing the central perception of dyspnea, decreasing anxiety, decreasing sensitivity to hypercapnia, reducing oxygen consumption, and improving cardiovascular hemodynamics. Systemic opioids also have a central antitussive effect and could be useful in treating chronic or refractory cough.

Data suggest that 80–95% of terminal cancer patients achieve significant relief of dyspnea using systemic opioids. Begin morphine at a low dose and slowly increase the dosage in opioid-naïve patients. Five mg of immediate-release oral morphine may suffice and can be dosed every 4 hours. A more conservative initial dosing of 2.5–5 mg morphine is recommended for elderly patients or patients with severe COPD as more potent opioid initiation is associated with adverse consequences with respect to respiratory suppression. Buccal and parenteral routes are useful for patients who are unable to take oral medications. Morphine 3 mg subcutaneously (SQ) every 4 hours regularly and 1.5 mg SQ every 1 hour for breakthrough dyspnea can also be used if the oral route is not available or reliable.

In the case above, the patient has COPD as well as lung cancer. He may benefit from a course of steroids. Give 8 mg of dexamethasone intravenously (IV) every day or 40 mg of oral prednisone daily. Continue steroids for up to 5 days and discontinue if you see no improvement in symptoms. Steroids may have the added benefit of decreasing bone pain secondary to metastatic disease. Benzodiazepines are a useful adjunct when concomitant anxiety is present. Chlorpromazine has been shown to decrease breathlessness without affecting ventilation or producing sedation. Consider a trial of chlorpromazine 7.5–25 mg orally or IV every 6–8 hours regularly or as needed for dyspnea.

Helium/oxygen (Heliox) is a potential attractive alternative for patients with dyspnea from partial airway obstruction. Heliox has a lower density than nitrogen/oxygen and promotes laminar flow, thus enabling greater alveolar ventilation at a given inspiratory pressure and diminishing the work of breathing. Other adjuvant therapies include antitussives such as gabapentin, benzonatate, and inhaled lidocaine. Mucolytics such as guaifenesin, nebulized acetylcysteine, and hypertonic saline may also have a role in relieving dyspnea.

In a patient who is actively dying, certain patterns of breathing are expected and often suggest that time is short, on the order of days to hours. These individuals may exhibit periods of tachypnea with very shallow respirations, open-mouth breathing ("guppy breathing"), and periods of apnea. The appearance of these changed respiratory patterns is not indicative of patient distress.

KEY POINTS TO REMEMBER

- Dyspnea is a subjective experience. The patient's report of dyspnea must not be discounted in the setting of normal vital signs and perception of easy work of breathing.
- Screening for dyspnea using a validated tool such as the Edmond Symptom Assessment Scale (ESAS) can be a useful tool for detecting symptoms.
- Opioids are the mainstay of treatment for dyspnea and should be used to relieve suffering.

Further Reading

Abernethy AP, McDonald CF, Frith PA, et al. Effect of palliative oxygen versus room air in relief of breathlessness in patients with refractory dyspnoea: a double-blind, randomised controlled trial. *Lancet.* 2010;376(9743):784–793.

Bausewein C, Booth S, Gysels M, Higginson IJ. Non-pharmacological interventions for breathlessness in advanced stages of malignant and non-malignant diseases. *Cochrane Database Syst Rev.* 2011;2:CD005623.

Currow D, Louw S, McCloud P, et al. Regular, sustained-release morphine for chronic breathlessness: a multicentre, double-blind, randomised, placebo-controlled trial. *Thorax.* 2020;75(1):50–56.

Curtis JR, Cook DJ, Sinuff T, et al. Noninvasive positive pressure ventilation in critical and palliative care settings: understanding the goals of therapy. *Crit Care Med.* 2007;35(3):932–939.

Haywood A, Duc J, Good P, et al. Systemic corticosteroids for the management of cancer-related breathlessness (dyspnoea) in adults. *Cochrane Database Syst Rev.* 2019;2:CD012704.

Hui D, Morgado M, Chisholm G, et al. High-flow oxygen and bilevel positive airway pressure for persistent dyspnea in patients with advanced cancer: a phase II randomized trial. *J Pain Symptom Manage.* 2013;46(4):463–473.

Jennings AL, Davies AN, Higgins JP, Gibbs JS, Broadley KE. A systematic review of the use of opioids in the management of dyspnoea. *Thorax.* 2002;57(11):939–944.

Kathiresan G, Clement RF, Sankaranarayanan MT. Dyspnea in lung cancer patients: a systematic review. *Lung Cancer (Auckl).* 2010;1:141–150. doi:10.2147/LCTT.S14426

9 Treating Dyspnea Through Reducing Malignant Pleural Effusion

Christine A. Crader

A 66-year-old female patient has presented to the emergency department with significantly increased dyspnea. She has a 4-year history of invasive ductal carcinoma of the left breast. She reported significant dyspnea with walking 5 feet from her bed to the toilet, which is an acute change for her over the past 5 days. She also has developed a dry cough over the past few weeks. There is increased dullness to percussion on the right approximately halfway up the chest, decreased expansion of the right chest, absent breath sounds halfway up on the right, with normal breath sounds and expansion on the left. No accessory muscle use for breathing was noted. Two-view chest x-ray revealed a large, right pleural effusion without mediastinal shift, mass, or infiltrate. After applying 4 L of oxygen via nasal cannula, her SpO_2 improved to 90%. She was admitted to the hospital for further management.

What do I do now?

When a patient with a known malignancy presents with increasing dyspnea and is found to have a pleural effusion, the natural instinct is to presume the effusion is also malignant. However, an attempt must be made to confirm the suspicion of malignant pleural effusion (MPE). The effusion could also be secondary to congestive heart failure (CHF) or a parapneumonic process, for instance, and those diagnoses would potentially lead to a very different treatment course for the patient. In women, the most common causes of MPE are breast and gynecologic malignancies, while in men, it is most commonly secondary to lung cancer. Men also have a higher incidence than women of MPE secondary to mesothelioma, likely related to a higher exposure to asbestos in the workplace. The prognosis for a patient diagnosed with a MPE is quite poor, with a median expected survival of 3–12 months, depending on the underlying malignancy. Shorter survival is associated with lung cancer and mesothelioma related MPEs, whereas breast cancer and lymphoma tend to impart a slightly longer median survival.[1] A pleural effusion causes the sensation of dyspnea due to a flattening or even inversion of the diaphragm on the side of the effusion. This leads to a restrictive defect in ventilation, which leads to a decrease in the lung volume and an increase in the work of breathing.

DIAGNOSIS

Our patient has presented with the common manifestations of a pleural effusion, increased dyspnea and a dry cough. In addition, the presence of fluid in the pleural space was confirmed on both chest x-ray and CT scan of the chest. To determine the etiology of the pleural effusion, a diagnostic thoracentesis must be undertaken. This is most commonly done with radiologic guidance, using ultrasound or CT. When the fluid is removed for diagnosis, it should be sent to the lab for protein, lactate dehydrogenase (LDH), glucose, total and differential cell counts, Gram stain, culture, and cytology. The patient should also have serum laboratory tests to measure LDH, protein, and glucose close to the time of the thoracentesis. An exudative effusion is defined by Light's criteria as having any one of the following features:

1. Ratio of fluid LDH to serum LDH > 0.6
2. Ratio of fluid protein to serum protein > 0.5

3. Pleural fluid LDH more than two-thirds of the upper limit of the lab's reference range of serum LDH.

Certainly, the findings of an exudative effusion in a patient with a known malignancy can give a strong indication that this effusion is likely to be malignant, but the confirmation will likely come with the cytology report. When the diagnostic thoracentesis is undertaken, it is wise to ask the performing physician to remove up to 1000 mL of fluid for patient comfort.

PROGNOSIS

Once the diagnosis of MPE has been confirmed based on cytology studies, one must assess the patient's prognosis in order to best choose the next step in controlling the MPE. There are currently two prognostic scores available that best predict survival with a MPE: the PROMISE score[2] and the LENT score.[3] The PROMISE score includes both biological and clinical information to estimate a patient's 3-month mortality, while the LENT score uses pleural fluid LDH, ECOG performance status, serum neutrophil-to-lymphocyte ratio, and tumor type to predict survival. The PROMISE score is calculated using data such as whether a patient has previously had radiation or chemotherapy, their score on the Eastern Cooperative Oncology Group (ECOG) Performance Status Scale, their white blood cell count and hemoglobin level, their C-reactive protein (CRP) level, and their type of cancer. A patient's prognosis has an impact on which treatment for the MPE might be most appropriate. Calculators for these scores are easily found on many phone apps.

Ninety percent of MPEs will recur after drainage, making assessment of prognosis important in determining the next appropriate intervention upon recurrence. Typically, once a MPE is confirmed, this places the patient in the category of having stage IV disease. In a patient with a very limited life expectancy, for instance less than 1 month, it is appropriate to consider as-needed thoracentesis based upon symptoms. In all other patients, the goal generally is to treat the patient in the way that provides the most comfort and the least time spent in the hospital or procedure area. These treatment options will be discussed now.

TREATMENT OPTIONS

There are several appropriate treatment options for MPE, and each one has indications for certain MPE situations, varying based on the patient's prognosis, presence of lung entrapment, and symptoms. The ultimate goal with any of these treatments is to achieve pleurodesis, which makes further accumulation of fluid in the pleural space difficult. Regardless of how large the effusion appears on imaging, if the patient is asymptomatic, there is no indication for any intervention other than clinical observation.

Thoracentesis

Because safer drainage alternatives have been developed, thoracentesis is becoming less favored for repetitive drainage of an MPE. Therapeutic thoracentesis, also known as therapeutic pleural aspiration, can be used as an initial intervention to determine whether the patient's symptoms will improve or resolve with aspiration. If there is improvement, guidance can be given to the patient for more definitive treatment. In a frail patient or a patient with a very limited life expectancy, if the MPE does not reaccumulate enough to cause symptoms, then no further intervention will have been necessary. This is a reasonable first-line approach in such a patient.[4] On chest x-ray, if there is evidence of shift of the mediastinum toward the side of the effusion, this indicates that there is a high likelihood of lung entrapment and that the patient would not benefit from thoracentesis. If the mediastinum shifts away from the effusion, this effusion would likely respond well to a therapeutic thoracentesis.

During a thoracentesis of any type, it is best to have the patient sitting in an upright position if at all possible. This minimizes the risk of hitting spleen or liver, as it allows the fluid to flow toward the posterior chest area. Using a catheter rather than a needle can also decrease the risk of pneumothorax. In addition, providing supplemental oxygen may help to minimize hypoxia related to the shifting ventilation and perfusion of the re-expanding lung.[1] Dyspnea can often be alleviated with the removal of 400–500 mL of fluid, although up to 1000–1500 mL should be able to be safely removed in one sitting. Fluid removal should be halted if the patient complains of chest pain or pressure as this may indicate the lung is not expanding freely. Coughing during thoracentesis is common and is not a reason to stop the procedure unless uncomfortable for the patient.[1]

Pleurodesis

Pleurodesis is the process of causing the visceral and parietal pleura of the lung to adhere together, thereby obliterating the pleural space. The expected outcome is that fluid will no longer be able to accumulate in the pleural space, thereby alleviating the symptoms related to a pleural effusion. The outcome of having pleural adhesion is desired in any patient who has recurrent MPE because when the parietal and visceral pleura adhere to each other, the space for recurrent fluid buildup is restricted or even eliminated.

There are several ways to accomplish pleural adhesion, both surgically and chemically. The goal is to irritate the pleural surfaces to cause inflammation and subsequently adherence to each other. Surgical pleurodesis is usually performed via a thoracotomy or video thoracoscopy. During this procedure, the surgeon will cause mechanical irritation to the pleura, often with a rough pad. Occasionally, the parietal pleura is surgically removed to cause adherence. Chemical pleurodesis is most often attempted via a chest tube, but now can also be performed via a tunneled pleural catheter (TPC). Once access to the pleural space has been ensured, a chemical such as talc, bleomycin, tetracycline, or povidone–iodine is introduced to cause the desired irritation and subsequently adherence of the pleura. This is known to be a painful procedure for the patient, and various studies have been done looking at the benefit of introducing lidocaine with the chemical. The chest tube is typically clamped after instillation of the chemical to allow it to have its full effect. Any fluid from the preexisting MPE should be drained before the pleurodesis is attempted, as having the lung fully re-inflated allows maximum apposition of the two pleural surfaces, leading to a higher rate of success.[1] There have been many studies done to determine if there is an ideal chemical sclerosing agent for pleurodesis, with studies ongoing. A talc slurry is the most cost-effective, widely available commercial agent used for attempts at pleurodesis. There has been research (the TIME1 trial) showing that concurrent use of nonsteroidal anti-inflammatory drugs (NSAIDs) for pain relief related to talc pleurodesis does not interfere with adherence of the pleural surfaces.[5] A recent study revealed that chemical pleurodesis can be safely effected via talc administered through a TPC.[6] The disadvantages to attempting pleurodesis using chemicals administered via a surgical procedure or a chest tube include several days of hospitalization, increased discomfort to the patient, the need for anesthesia in the case of a surgical procedure, and increased cost overall.

TPC

A TPC, also sometimes referred to as an indwelling pleural catheter, is typically placed with local anesthesia in an outpatient setting. These have been in use in the United States since the late 1990s. Unlike the procedures discussed previously for pleurodesis, a TPC can be used in a patient who appears to have trapped lung. These catheters can be left in for several months and in fact are the most cost-effective approach to managing an MPE in a patient whose life expectancy is predicted to be greater than 3 months. There is evidence that a TPC can relieve dyspnea from an MPE as well as talc pleurodesis with a talc slurry administered via chest tube.[7] After a TPC is placed, the patient can then have their effusion drained at home. If able, the patient can do it themselves, or a caregiver can be trained to drain the TPC when indicated. This obviates the need to go back and forth to the hospital or clinic to have the MPE drained. The ASAP trial investigated the optimal frequency of TPC drainage to achieve auto-pleurodesis. The researchers determined that draining the TPC on a daily basis led to more frequent auto-pleurodesis than draining the effusion every other day. When auto-pleurodesis is achieved, it is then possible to remove the TPC.[8] In looking at whether patients undergoing TPC versus talc pleurodesis via chest tube have a difference in hospital days post-procedure, the AMPLE study indicated that the patients with a TPC had significantly fewer days in the hospital in the 12 months post-procedure.[9] The risks related to TPCs include the following: (1) catheter malfunction and clogging, which may require an intervention such as flushing or instilling an agent to lyse adhesions, etc.; (2) pain; (3) infection; and (4) rarely, tumor invasion of the tunneled site.[1] Patients with a TPC can still receive palliative chemotherapy.

TABLE 9.1. **Summary of Interventions for MPE**

Intervention	Indications	Contraindications	Risks	Benefits
Thoracentesis/ therapeutic pleural aspiration	• Evidence of pleural fluid on imaging • Need to confirm malignant cells in fluid • Symptomatic dyspnea from MPE	Absolute: • Ipsilateral mediastinal shift Relative: • Coagulopathy • Agitated or uncooperative patient	Bleeding, pneumothorax, infection	• Minimally invasive • Almost universally available • Quick turnaround for results
Pleurodesis via chest tube with sclerosing agent	Recurrent accumulation of MPE	Inability to fully drain MPE prior to sclerosant instillation	Chest pain, bleeding, infection, fever, nausea, need for increased analgesia; usually requires hospital stay	Can resolve loculations
Surgical pleurodesis	• MPE with trapped lung • Loculated pleural fluid • Chylous effusion • Presence of a diaphragmatic defect	Absolute: • Inability to tolerate anesthesia Relative: • Coagulopathy • Palliative Performance Scale < 70 • Life expectancy <3 months	Bleeding, chest pain, infection, fever, nausea	Drainage of loculated MPE
TPC	• Recurrent MPE requiring drainage • Trapped lung with MPE	Life expectancy <3 months	Catheter malfunction or clogging; pain at tunnel site; tumor invasion of tunnel track; infection	Can be done on an outpatient basis; cost-effective; fewer hospital days
Systemic chemotherapy	Chemotherapy-sensitive malignancy with MPE	Poor performance status; lack of chemosensitive tumor	Length of time to effect; systemic side effects	Noninvasive procedure

Data from references 1 and 4.

Systemic Chemotherapy

In patients with a malignancy that may be responsive to systemic chemotherapy, particularly breast cancer and lymphoma, proceeding with that therapy would certainly be indicated on a palliative basis to help manage the MPE. It is appropriate to perform the diagnostic and if necessary therapeutic thoracentesis concurrently with beginning the chemotherapy in order to serve as a bridge until the systemic therapy is determined to be effective.

Table 9.1 provides a summary of interventions.

Now, with all of this knowledge fresh in our minds, let's return to our 66-year-old patient with the right-sided pleural effusion and known metastatic breast cancer. Our next step would be to proceed with a diagnostic thoracentesis, with pleural fluid being sent to the lab for LDH, protein, glucose, cell counts and differential, culture, and cytology. In an attempt to provide some immediate relief from her dyspnea, we would ask the physician performing the thoracentesis to remove up to 1 L of pleural fluid. Her response to this drainage will guide us as to our next steps. If her dyspnea is not relieved by a moderate- to large-volume thoracentesis, then we need to investigate for other causes of her dyspnea. If her dyspnea does improve, then we can make plans for attempting other interventions. If she has systemic chemotherapy that her breast cancer may respond to, this would be an appropriate next step. If not, or if after treatment with any chemotherapeutic agents she has a recurrence of her MPE, then we would consider having a TPC placed for daily drainage in the home.

KEY POINTS TO REMEMBER

- An MPE indicates a very poor prognosis in most cases.
- A TPC is as effective as a chest tube with talc slurry for causing auto-pleurodesis of an MPE.
- NSAIDs can be used for pain relief while attempting pleurodesis.
- Use of a chest tube or surgical intervention for pleurodesis results in more hospital days for patients with an MPE than having a TPC placed.
- Shift of the mediastinum away from the side of the effusion indicates it will most likely be amenable to thoracentesis.

Further Reading

Keshishyan S, Harris K. Asymptomatic malignant pleural effusion: to observe or to manage. *J Thoracic Dis*. 2017(supp 10):S1146–S1147.

References

1. Boka K, Soo Hoo GW. Pleural effusion. *Medscape*. December 28, 2018.
2. Psallidas I, Kanellakis NI, Gerry S, et al. Development and validation of response markers to predict survival and pleurodesis success in patients with malignant pleural effusion (PROMISE); a multicohort analysis. *Lancet Oncol*. 2018;19(7):930–939.
3. Clive AO, Kahan BC, Hooper CE, et al. Predicting survival in malignant pleural effusion: development and validation of the LENT prognostic score. *Thorax*. 2014;69:1098–1104.
4. McCracken DJ, Rahman NM. Management of malignant pleural effusion. *Clin Pulm Med*. 2018;25(6):215–219.
5. Rahman NM, Pepperell J, Rehal S, et al. Effect of opioids vs NSAIDs and larger vs smaller chest tube size on pain control and pleurodesis efficacy among patients with malignant pleural effusion: the TIME1 randomized clinical trial. *JAMA*. 2015;314:2641–2653.
6. Bhatnagar R, Keenan EK, Morley AJ, et al. Outpatient talc administration by indwelling pleural catheter for malignant effusion. *N Engl J Med*. 2018;378(14):1313–1322.
7. Davies HE, Mishra EK, Kahan BC, et al. Effect of an indwelling pleural catheter vs. chest tube and talc pleurodesis for relieving dyspnea in patients with malignant pleural effusion: the TIME2 randomized controlled trial. *JAMA*. 2012;307(22):2383–2389.
8. Wahidi MM, Reddy C, Yarmus L, et al. Randomized trial of pleural fluid drainage frequency in patients with malignant pleural effusions: the ASAP trial. *Am J Respir Crit Care Med*. 2017;195:1050–1057.
9. Thomas R, Fysh ETH, Smith NA, et al. Effect of an indwelling pleural catheter vs talc pleurodesis on hospitalization days in patients with malignant pleural effusion: the AMPLE randomized clinical trial. *JAMA*. 2017;318:1903–1912.

10 Treating Dyspnea in Lung Cancer with Noninvasive Ventilation

Vittoria Comellini and Stefano Nava

A 60-year-old woman was admitted to the hospital via the emergency department with acute hypoxemic respiratory failure. She has a history of lung cancer. She reported severe dyspnea (8/10 on the Borg scale) and nonproductive cough associated with fever with onset in the previous 2 days. Vital signs were as follows: temperature 38.3°, blood pressure 130/80, heart rate 128, respiratory rate 35. Lungs: diminished lung sounds, bibasilar crackles and expiratory wheeze, accessory muscle use, SpO_2 83% on oxygen (8 L/min) humidified nasal cannula. Chest x-ray showed hypodiaphania of the upper right lobe, referable to the known cancer, and new-onset bilateral infiltrates; no pleural effusions or signs referable to heart failure. The patient was treated with antibiotic and antipyretic therapy. Oxygen was administered through a high-flow nasal cannula with improvement of the PaO_2/FiO_2 ratio from arterial blood samples (from 130 to 180). However, significant dyspnea persisted, resulting in respiratory distress and severe anxiety.

What do I do now?

Dyspnea is a common, subjective, multidimensional, and distressing symptom, experienced by 19–51% of patients with advanced cancer, especially when they approach end of life.[1] While the prevalence of dyspnea has been reported to be as frequent as pain in people with lung cancer, less attention has been paid to the distress associated with breathlessness. Usually dyspnea and the associated anxiety are managed with pharmacological treatments, sometimes associated with psychosocial support. As cancer patients advance in their disease process, palliative therapies may be necessary for symptom relief. Both pharmacological and nonpharmacological treatments can be administered to assist patients and to improve the quality of their lives.

To the best of our knowledge, there are only two randomized controlled trials (RTCs) and no specific studies published on the topic of noninvasive ventilation (NIV) in lung cancer patients. However, as evidenced by the limited published trials, NIV seems to be a promising option for the treatment of cancer patients.[2]

In the present chapter we will deal only with patients affected by solid cancer, since patients with hematological ones respond to NIV in a different manner.[3]

NIV has not been applied systematically in patients with solid cancer, even when they experience an episode of acute respiratory failure (ARF). A possible explanation is that this technique is often considered to be a disproportionate intervention compared to life expectancy for cancer patients, including those suffering from lung cancer. However, even in this population we can identify potentially ideal candidates for NIV, as suggested by the latest guidelines published by the European Respiratory Society (ERS) and the American Thoracic Society (ATS).[4]

First of all, NIV can alleviate dyspnea due to respiratory muscle unloading. The intensity of dyspnea frequently worsens as the disease progresses, and patients and their families expect symptomatic relief of this devastating symptom. Clinicians often prescribe analgo-sedation and opioids, which is a highly effective treatment but one that has a number of potentially undesirable side effects, including respiratory depression and excessive sedation. Patients with advanced lung cancer may also experience dyspnea caused by fatigue and respiratory muscle wasting. NIV, administered intermittently or continuously, can be helpful to those patients who have respiratory muscle fatigue.[5] It is usually administered via nasal masks or less frequently with a helmet, possibly using a rotating strategy between the different interfaces. Two RCTs showed that NIV is effective in reducing breathlessness among patients with advanced cancer. Hui et al.[6] showed in a physiological short-term trial that treatment with NIV and high-flow humidified oxygen induced a similar improvement in dyspnea scores. In a larger multicenter study, Nava et al.[7] demonstrated a significantly greater reduction in breathlessness using NIV to treat patients with solid cancers, especially in the hypercapnic subgroup of patients. Interestingly, the latter investigators showed that NIV might reduce the dose of morphine necessary to palliate dyspnea, maintaining better cognitive function. Moreover, NIV had a similar rate of acceptance by patients compared with those treated with oxygen therapy (~60%). A similar use of NIV in palliative care was indicated by the Task Force of the Society of Critical Care Medicine.[8] Therefore, offering NIV to dyspneic patients for palliation in the setting of advanced or terminal lung cancer can alleviate breathlessness and ensure comfort while dying. From an ethical perspective, clinicians should be aware that, in this context, NIV would be considered effective if it improves breathlessness without causing other troubling consequences, such as mask discomfort, inability to communicate, or unduly prolonging life. A crucial point in clinical practice and research is therefore identifying which patients will benefit most from NIV and who would not, avoiding in the latter case the use of futile mechanical support.

A second important field of application of NIV in the oncologic and palliative setting is the treatment of ARF episodes, and the dyspnea and respiratory distress associated with them. Contrary to popular belief, ARF episodes are by far the most common reason for cancer patients to be admitted to an intensive care unit (ICU).[9] The occurrence of ARF often represents the terminal phase of the disease and it is related to a dramatically high mortality rate, independently of the type of cancer.[10–13] Indeed, the overall survival of cancer patients admitted to the ICU is very disappointing, especially in the subgroup of patients requiring mechanical ventilation, in whom the mortality rate has been reported to exceed 80%.[9,10,12,13] As a consequence, cancer patients with severe respiratory failure are frequently denied admission to an ICU. This is mainly due to the fact that intubation and mechanical ventilation are both strong predictors of mortality, particularly in the subset of patients who are not receiving chemotherapy or radiotherapy because of the advanced stage of their disease.[10] Therefore, as previously stated, based on studies reporting limited survival at considerable costs in such patients, oxygen therapy and morphine often represent the only attempt to improve oxygenation and/or relieve dyspnea.[10,14] Most patients with advanced or end-stage lung cancer receiving only palliative care have a do-not-intubate (DNI) order. Even when formal, prospective decisions on this aspect have not been made, these patients do not receive endotracheal intubation because of the low survival rates compared to the considerable costs. However, patients may be affected by comorbid conditions and at some point may develop ARF that is not necessarily related to the site or progression of the lung cancer. For example, a consistent proportion of cancer patients are smokers or ex-smokers; thus, they frequently also have chronic pulmonary disease or cardiac disease, and the occurrence of an acute exacerbation of the underlying disease, leading to ARF, is relatively common. It's important to underline that these episodes of ARF are not necessarily related to cancer progression; in some cases, they may have a potentially treatable and reversible cause such as cardiogenic pulmonary edema, pulmonary infection, or an acute exacerbation of chronic obstructive pulmonary disease (COPD) or atelectasis. Even though most of these ARF episodes may be promptly reversible if adequately treated, these patients often do not receive any form of ventilatory support because they have an underlying tumor. In this second scenario, NIV represents a salvage therapy with the goal of surviving the hospitalization, even and paradoxically when survival is not necessarily a primary goal. The literature of the last decade shows us encouraging data that document that NIV may have a protective effect from mortality even in critically ill cancer patients. NIV has been used as a treatment of ARF in COPD patients with a DNI order.[15] In one case–control study comparing the efficacy of NIV versus invasive mechanical ventilation (IMV) in patients with different types of malignancies,[16] mortality has improved when NIV was applied. Previous experiences have shown that the use of NIV in patients with end-stage solid cancer complicated by ARF is feasible and useful in providing rapid improvement in dyspnea, arterial blood gas results, and other physiological variables.[17] These studies showed that NIV has a favorable short-term outcome and helps cancer patients to overcome an acute phase of illness, prolonging their lives. NIV can provide some additional time, for example, for life closure tasks to be completed (e.g., saying goodbye to relatives and friends or solving some administrative issues). NIV represents a generally well-tolerated and valid tool for patients with cancer; it alleviates respiratory distress and lessens dyspnea while preserving the patient's autonomy, verbal communication, and eating. Nevertheless, most clinicians are unclear about the goals of care, and it has been highlighted that NIV may be inappropriate in this context because of an increased use of medical resources, prolongation of the dying process, and intensification of suffering.[8] Clinicians have to be very careful and refrain from prolonging survival in a futile manner in patients whose death is inevitable. NIV should thus be proposed in lung cancer patients who still have a therapeutic plan and who present with a reversible cause of ARF. Because we lack data from RCTs, we must first identify and propose this ventilatory technique only on the basis of an individual approach, taking into account the patient's clinical condition and prior expressed wishes and/or the presence of advance directives. Indeed, when considering what therapies are best, it is important to discuss the goals of care with the patient and family. Although laws differ across countries, during the last decades legislation has made progress regarding the possibility for the patient to prepare advance directives while still competent, and patients with cancer are now more involved in end-of-life decision-making. The best approach suggested should therefore be based on the active participation of the patient, explaining to them the goals of care and emphasizing the importance of information and communication with family members and caregivers.

Another important aspect is where to treat the lung cancer patient with NIV. The large majority of patients are treated in a protected environment like the ICU or a specialized respiratory ICU (RICU), where adequately trained and competent medical, physiotherapeutic, or nursing staff members are available for the application of the technique. However, as shown by Cuomo et al.,[17] it is feasible to treat cancer patients with NIV outside the ICUs, for example in medical departments or in palliative care units.

KEY POINTS TO REMEMBER

- The prevalence of dyspnea has been reported to be as frequent as pain in people with lung cancer.
- Most end-stage lung patients do not receive any form of ventilatory support, since they are considered terminally ill.
- Noninvasive ventilation (NIV) may act as a palliative tool, improving dyspnea and reducing the need for opioids.
- High-flow humidified oxygen may be an alternative to NIV in this setting, but this should be further explored in RTCs.
- Despite the ERS/ATS guidelines recommending the use of NIV as a palliative treatment in solid cancer patients, the team in charge of its application should be trained and experienced in the delivery of this form of treatment.
- The patient has the right to stop NIV at any time, while the clinician may consider stopping it when tolerance is poor or when dyspnea does not improve.

References

1. Beckles MA, Spiro SG, Colice GL, Rudd RM. Initial evaluation of the patient with lung cancer: symptoms, signs, laboratory tests, and paraneoplastic syndromes. *Chest*. 2003;123:97S–104S. doi:10.1378/chest.123.1_suppl.97S
2. Quill CM, Quill TE. Palliative use of noninvasive ventilation: navigating murky waters. *J Palliat Med*. 2014;17:657–661. doi:10.1089/jpm.2014.0010
3. Vadde R, Pastores SM. Management of acute respiratory failure in patients with hematological malignancy. *J Intensive Care Med*. 2016;31:627–641. doi:10.1177/0885066615601046
4. Rochwerg B, Brochard L, Elliott MW, et al. Official ERS/ATS clinical practice guidelines: noninvasive ventilation for acute respiratory failure. *Eur Respir J*. 2017;50:1–20. doi:10.1183/13993003.02426-2016
5. Pisani L, Hill NS, Pacilli AMG, Polastri M, Nava S. Management of dyspnea in the terminally ill. *Chest*. 2018;154:925–934. doi:10.1016/j.chest.2018.04.003
6. Hui D, Morgado M, Chisholm G, et al. High-flow oxygen and bilevel positive airway pressure for persistent dyspnea in patients with advanced cancer: a phase II randomized trial. *J Pain Symptom Manage*. 2013;46:463–473. doi:10.1016/j.jpainsymman.2012.10.284
7. Nava S, Ferrer M, Esquinas A, et al. Palliative use of non-invasive ventilation in end-of-life patients with solid tumours: a randomised feasibility trial. *Lancet Oncol*. 2013;14:219–227. doi:10.1016/S1470-2045(13)70009-3

8. Curtis JR, Cook DJ, Sinuff T, et al. Noninvasive positive pressure ventilation in critical and palliative care settings: understanding the goals of therapy. *Crit Care Med.* 2007;35:932–939. doi:10.1097/01.CCM.0000256725.73993.74

9. Blot F, Guiguet M, Nitenberg G, Leclercq B, Gachot B, Escudier B. Prognostic factors for neutropenic patients in an intensive care unit: respective roles of underlying malignancies and acute organ failures. *Eur J Cancer Part A.* 1997;33:1031–1037. doi:10.1016/S0959-8049(97)00042-7

10. Kress JP, Christenson J, Pohlman AS, Linkin DR, Hall JB. Outcomes of critically ill cancer patients in a university hospital setting. *Am J Respir Crit Care Med.* 1999;1160:1957–196. doi:10.1164/ajrccm.160.6.9812055

11. Rubenfeld GD, Crawford SW. Withdrawing life support from mechanically ventilated recipients of bone marrow transplants: a case for evidence-based guidelines. *Ann Intern Med.* 1996;125:625–633. doi:10.7326/0003-4819-125-8-199610150-00001

12. Groeger JS, Lemeshow S, Price K, et al. Multicenter outcome study of cancer patients admitted to the intensive care unit: a probability of mortality model. *J Clin Oncol.* 1998;16:761–770. doi:10.1200/JCO.1998.16.2.761

13. Kroschinsky F, Weise M, Illmer T, et al. Outcome and prognostic features of intensive care unit treatment in patients with hematological malignancies. *Intensive Care Med.* 2002;28:1294–1300. doi:10.1007/s00134-002-1420-5

14. Faber-Langendoen K, Caplan AL, McGlave PB. Survival of adult bone marrow transplant patients receiving mechanical ventilation: a case for restricted use. *Bone Marrow Transplant.* 1993;12:501–507.

15. Chu CM, Chan VL, Wong IWY, Leung WS, Lin AWN, Cheung KF. Noninvasive ventilation in patients with acute hypercapnic exacerbation of chronic obstructive pulmonary disease who refused endotracheal intubation. *Crit Care Med.* 2004;32:372–377. doi:10.1097/01.CCM.0000108879.86838.4F

16. Azoulay E, Alberti C, Bornstain C, et al. Improved survival in cancer patients requiring mechanical ventilatory support: impact of noninvasive mechanical ventilatory support. *Crit Care Med.* 2001;29:519–525. doi:10.1097/00003246-200103000-00009

17. Cuomo A, Delmastro M, Ceriana P, et al. Noninvasive mechanical ventilation as a palliative treatment of acute respiratory failure in patients with end-stage solid cancer. *Palliat Med.* 2004;18:602–610. doi:10.1191/0269216304pm933oa

11 Palliative Care for Infants with Bronchopulmonary Dysplasia

Christine A. Fortney and Jodi A. Ulloa

An extremely premature female infant who was delivered by emergency cesarean section for fetal distress remains in the neonatal intensive care unit (NICU) where she has been hospitalized since birth. She is now 4 months old (39 weeks post-menstrual age) and has failed multiple attempts to extubate from conventional mechanical ventilation (CMV) to nasal continuous positive airway pressure (NCPAP) over the last several weeks. Chest x-ray shows severe bronchopulmonary dysplasia (BPD) and she remains on CMV settings with a 60–75% oxygen requirement, increased work of breathing accompanied by frequent desaturation episodes, and below-expected anthropometric growth parameters. She frequently requires sedation with medications when distressed, which impairs her ability to interact with family or caregivers and has resulted in a delay achieving appropriate developmental milestones. She is receiving full enteral nutrition delivered via oral gastric tube.

What do I do now?

I n this infant who has developed a complex chronic condition as a result
of her prematurity, there are several concerns about her long-term development. She continues to experience respiratory distress requiring CMV
and sedation, which is affecting her growth and development, as well as her
ability to bond with her family.

Infants with respiratory distress syndrome (RDS) are vulnerable at birth
to significant lung injury because of damage to developing lungs by the
application of medical treatment necessary to sustain life. BPD remains
the most common chronic lung disease in infants born before 30 weeks of
gestation. BPD is classified as the need for supplemental oxygen and level
of respiratory support at 36 weeks post-menstrual age. A diagnosis of BPD
can prolong an infant's hospital stay for many months, or even years, while
the infant receives continued treatment for management of their condition,
and also places them at risk for significant pulmonary sequelae throughout
infancy and childhood and even into adulthood. Primarily, optimal respiratory support provides adequate ventilation/perfusion matching to allow for
the appropriate development and growth of the lungs and brain of the infant and to promote interaction with their environmental surroundings and
caregivers. However, only the prevention of premature birth is the primary
intervention currently recommended to prevent the development of BPD.

The extremely premature infant's comfort and quality of life, as well as
family involvement in their care, should be a focus of the treatment plan,
ideally from admission to the NICU but certainly from the time of diagnosis of BPD, and should continue throughout their illness trajectory. Not
only are these infants at high risk for poor long-term outcomes, but their
parents are also at risk for depression and anxiety, with up to 30% of NICU
parents experiencing issues with their mental health in the year following
the birth of the infant.

PRIMARY PALLIATIVE CARE IN THE NICU

Because advances in neonatal care now allow for the survival of many infants
who would have previously died from their conditions, concerns regarding
poor prognosis and quality of life necessitate the early introduction of palliative care to provide adequate support to infants and their families to reduce symptoms and suffering, improve quality of life, mitigate distress, and

support complex decision-making. Neonatal nurses; NICU psychologists; respiratory therapists; pharmacists; speech, physical, and occupational therapists; lactation consultants; social workers; chaplains; trainees of all disciplines; neonatal nurse practitioners; and physicians should strive to provide primary palliative care to infants and their families. This care begins with the inclusion of basic management of the infant's pain and symptoms as well as parental anxiety and depression, and open and honest discussions about prognosis, goals of treatment, and resuscitation goals of care. Individualized care plans may then be developed in conjunction with the family to support the specific needs of the infant.

Symptom assessment in infants can be difficult because they are non-verbal, their symptoms may have multiple meanings (e.g., crying could be the result of pain, hunger, a soiled diaper, or a need to be held), and there is a lack of valid and reliable measurement tools available for infants. Ongoing assessment of symptoms that indicate levels of infant pain are measured on pain scales completed by NICU staff; these tools vary by age and institutional preferences. Unfortunately, respiratory distress symptoms experienced by infants with severe BPD frequently mimic pain symptoms scored on these tools, with increased vital signs, crying, and increased work of breathing further complicating the management of these infants.

Infant respiratory symptoms are often treated with bronchodilators, inhaled corticosteroids, and oral diuretics, while pain, agitation, and irritability associated with air hunger can be managed with opioids (e.g., morphine) and benzodiazepines (e.g., lorazepam), which act on the central nervous system to produce a calming effect. It is important to note that these medications may decrease respiratory drive, so providers and parents should establish clear goals of care. Since many symptoms in infants remain unresolved and complex, a palliative care service that includes healthcare providers who are specially trained in palliative care with specialty expertise in neonatal care can be consulted for additional options to further treat the infant and family. However, the palliative care team should be introduced well in advance of a transition to an end-of-life (EOL) scenario to achieve maximum benefit for the infant and family. This combination of primary and consultative palliative care that starts early during the hospital admission allows for the integration of palliative care into routine NICU care to provide simultaneous delivery of services that are tailored to meet the specific needs of the infant and family. Palliative care can and should be delivered in conjunction with curative therapies until the infant either no longer responds to curative therapy and transitions to EOL care or improves to a level where palliative care is no longer required.

Palliative care can also be transitioned to the home setting. The number of infants with BPD discharged home from the NICU on oxygen increases every year, and infants and families need continued support to minimize symptoms, prevent and treat suffering, and emphasize quality of life outside of the hospital setting. Parental involvement in the care of an infant with BPD, starting in the NICU and continued at home, can positively affect the course of the disease and the overall development of an infant.

This infant was initially managed using a primary palliative care approach in the NICU. The entire NICU healthcare team worked together to stabilize the infant and support the family. Ongoing conversations with the parents provided guidance to the team about their preferences (cultural, spiritual, emotional) and treatment goals of care for their daughter. When the infant's symptoms did not resolve using standard therapies, the hospital's palliative care service was consulted to provide additional options for symptom management and family support, as well as to revisit the treatment goals of care. The infant ultimately was able to make enough progress to be discharged to home, despite an ongoing complex chronic condition. The palliative care service assisted in transitioning the infant and her family to home-based palliative care that could provide ongoing support while the delivery of outpatient care services continued through neonatal follow-up and complex care teams.

KEY POINTS TO REMEMBER

- BPD remains the most common chronic lung disease in infants born before 30 weeks gestational age.
- A diagnosis of BPD can prolong an infant's hospital stay for many months, or even years, while the infant receives continued treatment for management of their condition.
- Early provision of palliative care can help minimize symptoms, prevent and treat suffering, and emphasize quality of life while emphasizing the specific needs of the patient and family.

- Palliative care can and should be delivered in conjunction with curative therapies until the infant either no longer responds to curative therapy and transitions to EOL care or improves to a level where palliative care is no longer required.
- A combination of primary and consultative palliative care started early in admission allows for the integration of palliative care services into routine NICU care to allow simultaneous instead of sequential delivery of palliative care that may also extend to the home setting.

Further Reading

Baron I, Rey-Casserly C. Extremely preterm birth outcomes: a review of four decades of cognitive research. *Neuropsychol Rev.* 2010; 20:430–452.

Baughcum AE, Fortney CA, Winning A, et al. Perspectives from bereaved parents on improving end of life care in the NICU. *Clin Pract Pediatr Psychol.* 2017;5(4):392–403.

Davidson L, Berkelhamer S. Bronchopulmonary dysplasia: chronic lung disease of infancy and long-term pulmonary outcomes. *J Clin Med.* 2017; 6(4):9–20.

Fortney CA, Campbell ML. Development and content validity of a respiratory distress observation scale—infant. *J Palliat Med.* 2020;23(6):838–841.

Kair L, Leonard D, Anderson J. Bronchopulmonary dysplasia. *Pediatr Rev.* 2012; 33:255–261.

Lau R, Crump T, Brousseau D, et al. Parent preferences regarding home oxygen use for infants with bronchopulmonary dysplasia. *J Pediatr.* 2019;213(October):30–37.

Logan JW, Lynch S, Curtiss J, Shepherd E. Clinical phenotypes and management concepts for severe, established bronchopulmonary dysplasia. *Pediatr Resp Rev.* 2019; 31:58–63.

Marc-Aurele KL, English NK. Primary palliative care in neonatal intensive care. *Semin Perinatol.* 2017;41:133–139.

12 Reducing Dyspnea by Treating Ascites

Habib A. Khan

A 65-year-old female with stage IV ovarian cancer
was sent to the emergency department (ED) from her
oncologist's office for difficulty breathing, early satiety,
abdominal pressure, and weakness for 4 days. Patient
states that her dyspnea gets worse when she lies
down flat, and she has started to sleep in a recliner
over the last 2 days. She feels she cannot take a deep
breath, and whenever she tries to, her abdominal
discomfort gets worse. Her appetite is fair, but she
gets full after eating only a few bites. Her disease
has progressed in the last year with metastasis to
the brain, lungs, and peritoneum and worsening of
her liver metastasis. She is cachectic, sitting up on
the exam bed with heart rate of 96, respiratory rate
of 24, and shallow breathing. She also has flank
fullness, abdominal distention, fluid thrill, and shifting
dullness. An abdominal ultrasound showed severe
ascites with no loculations.

What do I do now?

Ascites is the pathological accumulation of fluid in the peritoneal cavity. The most common cause (85%) of ascites is cirrhosis.[1] Other causes include cancers, heart failure, Budd–Chiari syndrome, or massive liver metastases leading to portal hypertension.[1,2] The most common cancers associated with ascites are adenocarcinomas of the ovary, breast, colon, lung, liver, and pancreas. In addition, lymphoma can be complicated by chylous ascites. The reported median survival after a diagnosis of malignancy-related ascites ranges from 1 to 4 months,[3] except for ovarian and breast cancers, in which survival can be longer if anticancer treatments are available. Patients with non-ovarian cancer (including effusion lymphoma) have a particularly poor prognosis, with an expected survival of less than 3 months.[3]

SYMPTOMS

Symptoms of ascites may include weight gain; fatigue; early satiety; abdominal pain, discomfort, and distention; dyspnea; and reduced mobility. The time course over which the distention develops depends upon the etiology of the ascites—for example, ascites due to trauma (bloody ascites) can develop over the course of days, while malignant ascites can take months to accumulate.

DIAGNOSIS

Diagnosis is usually made based on the patient's history, physical examination, and ultrasonography. Physical examination will show abdominal distention, fluid thrill/wave (the patient or a colleague push their hands in midline and the examiner taps one flank while feeling for a wave or thrill in the other flank), shifting dullness (a change in the location of dullness to percussion when the patient is turned due to movement of the ascites), flank fullness/dullness, and sometimes signs related to the underlying cause of the ascites, such as stigmata of cirrhosis. Ultrasound can confirm the presence of ascites and demonstrate if the fluid is loculated in discrete areas of the peritoneal cavity, which is important once a decision is made to drain it.

ETIOLOGY

After diagnosis, the next step is to look for the cause. This typically includes blood work for serum albumin and a paracentesis to evaluate the ascitic fluid WBC count, albumin, protein, and cytology. The serum–ascites albumin gradient (SAAG) can be easily calculated to determine the etiology of ascites by identifying the presence of portal hypertension:[1]

SAAG = (serum albumin concentration) – (ascitic fluid albumin concentration)

A SAAG > 1.1 g/dL indicates portal hypertension, with 96.7% accuracy. It is usually seen in patients with cirrhosis, hepatic congestion, congestive heart failure (CHF), or portal vein thrombosis. A SAAG < 1.1 g/dL indicates no portal hypertension, with 96.7% accuracy. It is usually seen in peritoneal carcinomatosis, an infectious process of the peritoneum, nephrotic syndrome, or malnutrition/hypoalbuminemia.

Cytological evaluation is approximately 96.7% sensitive in cases of peritoneal carcinomatosis[2] but is not helpful in the detection of other types of malignant ascites.

TREATMENT

Treatment of ascites is usually aimed at its cause, like treating heart failure or surgical debulking and chemotherapy in advanced ovarian cancer. If that fails, then treatment is aimed at alleviating symptoms in palliative care, just like any other disease process treatment. Dietary restrictions are not warranted so as not to impair the patient's quality of life. Diuretics and peritoneovenous shunts (PVSs) are also tried. Therapeutic paracentesis is the primary treatment for peritoneal carcinomatosis. Peritoneal ports and catheters can be considered for patients who are intolerant of repeated paracenteses.

Tumor-Targeted Treatment
Depending in part upon the tumor type, specific tumor-targeted treatments may be appropriate to treat ascites.

Debulking, Chemotherapy, and Vascular Endothelial Growth Factor (VEGF) Inhibitors

Patients with ovarian, fallopian tube, or peritoneal carcinoma might be operative candidates at the time of presentation. Surgical debulking followed by chemotherapy or neoadjuvant chemotherapy[4] can be done to help improve symptoms. Most women with chemotherapy-resistant epithelial ovarian cancer who develop ascites may obtain symptomatic relief with systemic administration of VEGF, although the evidence is limited

Hyperthermic Intraperitoneal Chemotherapy (HIPEC)

Patients with peritoneal mesothelioma, diffuse peritoneal adenomucinosis (pseudomyxoma peritonei), and possibly selected patients with isolated peritoneal carcinomatosis from appendiceal or colorectal adenocarcinoma may benefit from aggressive cytoreductive therapy or tumor debulking combined with infusion of warmed chemotherapy (performed by a surgical oncologist) into the peritoneal cavity for a short period of time. Recovery from HIPEC with cytoreductive surgery (CRS) can take 3–6 months, so it is typically reserved for patients whose tumors are associated with a longer survival. For patients with anticipated shorter survivals, HIPEC without CRS can be done laparoscopically (and is therefore associated with less morbidity) with high rates of ascites control. Intraperitoneal administration of anticancer drugs enables direct contact of extremely high drug concentrations with the malignant lesions within the peritoneal cavity. However, while some studies suggest promise,[5-7] no role has been established for intraperitoneal rather than intravenous administration of cytotoxic chemotherapy for patients with malignancy-related ascites and a tumor other than epithelial ovarian cancer.

Diuretics

Diuretics may be effective in some patients with malignancy-related ascites, particularly in those with portal hypertension such as from massive liver metastases. The two commonly used diuretics are furosemide and spironolactone, and doses are adjusted in a ratio of 100 mg/day of spironolactone and 40 mg/day of oral furosemide to achieve natriuresis and weight loss.

Vascular Shunts

PVSs (LeVeen or Denver shunt) channel ascitic fluid back into the circulation via the superior vena cava. The best response to PVS (only about 50%) is in ovarian cancers, breast cancers, or diuretic-resistant ascites. This intervention is recommended only in patients with a life expectancy of 1–4 months. Due to the high rate of complications, PVS is rarely done today.

A transjugular intrahepatic portosystemic shunt (TIPS) between the portal vein and the hepatic vein is designed to reduce portal hypertension and improve sodium balance. Most patients with malignant ascites do not have portal hypertension, although TIPS might be helpful in the occasional cancer with evidence of increased portal pressures (SAAG > 1.1).

Paracentesis

Therapeutic paracentesis is the mainstay of treatment for peritoneal carcinomatosis that is not due to ovarian cancer. Paracentesis can provide immediate relief of symptoms in up to 90% of patients with as little as a few liters of fluid removed.[8,9] Large-volume abdominal paracentesis (LVP) is usually needed every 1–2 weeks, although the frequency should be guided by the patient's symptoms (e.g., distention, shortness of breath, early satiety). The goal in patients with malignancy-related ascites is to efficiently drain all readily removable fluid.

Drainage of uncomplicated large-volume ascites (4–6 L/session) can be done safely and quickly in the outpatient setting or at the hospital bedside; ultrasound guidance is necessary only when there is loculated fluid. Unlike patients with ascites due to portal hypertension, patients with malignancy-related ascites can have large volumes of fluid (up to 21 L) removed without fear of hemodynamic sequelae, including circulatory failure.[10] For patients undergoing LVP for malignancy-related ascites, using colloid replacement with intravenous albumin is not necessary. For hospice patients with symptomatic recurrent ascites requiring frequent LVP, home-based paracentesis may also be an option, provided a qualified physician, nurse practitioner, or physician's assistant is available to perform the procedure.[11] Tunneled indwelling peritoneal catheters are an alternative, permanent drainage system that allows patients to control symptoms in the home setting for recurrent LVP.

Drainage Catheters

Physical symptoms, plus the need to travel to an office for repeat procedures, can pose a significant burden[8] on the patient and caregivers, affecting quality of life. Peritoneal ports or indwelling tunneled catheter drainage systems can be placed that permit removal of the fluid at home by a visiting nurse, the patient, or a family member to avoid repeated needle insertions and extra visits to doctors. Although leakage around the insertion site and infection is a potential complication,[12,13] the overall risk appears to be low[14] and infections can often be treated without removing the catheter. Contraindications include single or multifocal loculated pockets of ascites, peritonitis, or uncorrected coagulopathy.[15]

There are two main types of catheters available, pigtail and tunneled. Pigtail catheters are prone to complications and are thus rarely used. Tunneled catheters, used conventionally for peritoneal dialysis, are placed under ultrasound or fluoroscopic guidance. The risk of infection is lowered by promoting scarring around an antibiotic-impregnated Dacron cuff in subcutaneous tissue. Complications are reduced by daily drainage for the first 2 weeks of cuff healing. These catheters are used in patients with a life expectancy of at least 1 month. The timing of placement for malignant ascites is empirical, although usually it is considered after a patient has had at least two prior LVPs.[2,9] The same considerations are relevant for nonmalignant ascites; however, due to survival and infection concerns, many clinicians limit the off-label use for nonmalignant ascites to patients with an anticipated survival of less than 2 months. Due to the cost of the initial procedure, catheter placement is often performed prior to hospice enrollment.

In the absence of successful treatment of the tumor itself, peritoneal implants continue to form, and as the implants adhere to previously successful paracentesis sites, performing successful paracentesis can become increasingly difficult. Image guidance can help in this setting. Eventually, the fluid becomes more solid and the patient may develop bowel obstruction, which can be fatal.

Considering the above information, let's get back to our patient, who has stage IV ovarian cancer with metastasis to the peritoneum, liver, brain, and lungs. She is experiencing progressive decline and is not appropriate for more definitive cancer treatment. At this stage her life expectancy is estimated to range from 1 to 4 months. She has had six paracenteses done in the last 2 years, with two in the past 2 weeks. With consistent clinical decline and failing paracenteses, a tunneled catheter can be placed at this time, and this patient can then be enrolled in hospice. A tunneled catheter will reduce her visits to the doctor and improve her quality of life; she or a family member, caregiver, or hospice nurse can drain it at home whenever she is symptomatic.

KEY POINTS TO REMEMBER

- Consider diuretics for patients with a SAAG > 1.
- For patients who require repeated paracentesis and have a prognosis of 1–3 months, consider tunneled catheters to decrease office visits and improve quality of life.
- If ultrasound shows the formation of loculations or pockets, then paracentesis should be done under ultrasound guidance.
- For palliative paracentesis, colloid replacement and diet restrictions are not recommended so as not to impair the patient's quality of life.

References

1. Runyon BA, Montano AA, Akriviadis EA, Antillon MR, Irving MA, McHutchison JG. The serum-ascites albumin gradient is superior to the exudate-transudate concept in the differential diagnosis of ascites, *Ann Intern Med.* 1992;117(3):215–220.
2. Runyon BA, Hoefs JC, Morgan TR. Ascitic fluid analysis in malignancy-related ascites. *Hepatology.* 1988;8(5):1104–1109.
3. Ayantunde AA, Parsons SL. Pattern and prognostic factors in patients with malignant ascites: a retrospective study. *Ann Oncol.* 2007;18(5):945–949.
4. Schumacher DL, Saclarides TJ, Staren ED. Peritoneovenous shunts for palliation of the patient with malignant ascites. *Ann Surg Oncol.* 1994;1(5):378–381.
5. Cannistra SA. Cancer of the ovary. *N Engl J Med* 2004;351:2519–2529.
6. Ng T, Pagliuca A, Mufti GJ. Intraperitoneal rituximab: an effective measure to control recurrent abdominal ascites due to non-Hodgkin's lymphoma. *Ann Hematol.* 2002;81(7):405–406.
7. Randle RW, Swett KR, Swords DS, et al. Efficacy of cytoreductive surgery with hyperthermic intraperitoneal chemotherapy in the management of malignant ascites. *Ann Surg Oncol.* 2014;21(5):1474–1479.

8. Becker G, Galandi D, Blum HE. Malignant ascites: systematic review and guideline for treatment. *Eur J Cancer*. 2006;42(5):589–597.
9. Saif MW, Siddiqui IA, Sohail MA. Management of ascites due to gastrointestinal malignancy. *Ann Saudi Med*. 2009;29(5):369–377.
10. Cruikshank DP, Buchsbaum HJ. Effects of rapid paracentesis: cardiovascular dynamics and body fluid composition. *JAMA*. 1973;225(11):1361–1362.
11. Zama IN, Edgar M. Management of symptomatic ascites in hospice patients with paracentesis: a case series report. *Am J Hosp Palliat Care*. 2012;29(5):405–408.
12. O'Neill MJ, Weissleder R, Gervais DA, Hahn PF, Mueller PR. Tunneled peritoneal catheter placement under sonographic and fluoroscopic guidance in the palliative treatment of malignant ascites. *AJR Am J Roentgenol*. 2001;177(3):615–618.
13. Savin MA, Kirsch MJ, Romano WJ, Wang SK, Arpasi PJ, Mazon CD. Peritoneal ports for treatment of intractable ascites. *J Vasc Interv Radiol*. 2005;16(3):363–368.
14. Wong BC, Cake L, Kachuik L, Amjadi K. Indwelling peritoneal catheters for managing malignancy-associated ascites. *J Palliat Care*. 2015;31(4):243–249.
15. Tapping CR, Ling L, Razack A. PleurX drain use in the management of malignant ascites: safety, complications, long-term patency and factors predictive of success. *Br J Radiol*. 2012;85(1013):623–628.

13 Panting for Breath in End-Stage Dementia

Hermien W. Goderie-Plomp,

Carole Parsons, David R. Mehr, and

Jenny T. van der Steen

You are summoned to the nursing home bed of an 82-year-old man. He is clearly experiencing respiratory distress with a respiratory rate of 33. He is somnolent but reacts to touch and speech; his breathing is audible. On auscultation, lungs give soft sounds, with diminished breath sounds in the right basal field and crackles in all other fields. Previously, he required support in his daily functioning in almost every domain due to his advanced Lewy body dementia, with a Barthel score of 15/100. Medications include macrogol 1 sachet/day, paracetamol 1000 mg three times daily, acetylsalicylic acid 80 mg/day, and enalapril 10 mg daily, with no allergies.

The family wants you to act; they can't stand to see their father this uncomfortable. Previously a do-not-resuscitate status was agreed upon, but no further discussions were held on treatment wishes, hospital or hospice admissions, artificial fluids or nutrition, or other end-of-life wishes.

What do I do now?

The differential diagnosis of dyspnea in patients with advanced dementia is broad, including, among others, pneumonia, pulmonary edema due to heart failure, pulmonary embolism, hyperventilation, exacerbation of chronic obstruction pulmonary disease (COPD), Kussmaul ventilation due to acidosis with hyperglycemia, and severe obstipation with a resulting elevated diaphragm. Also, in the nursing home setting, the available diagnostic tools are often very limited and the impact of tests on the patient's well-being must be taken into consideration. Patient medical history is not always present or trustworthy; medical history from the nursing staff is often fragmented. Neither x-ray nor ultrasound imaging is available on site; auscultation gives limited information as the patient cannot follow instructions and breathing sounds are often very soft. A point-of-care C-Reactive Protein (CRP) measurement can be helpful, as is a point-of-care glucose measurement. Other blood diagnostics often take over 24 hours to yield results.

PNEUMONIA

Given the nurses' reports and the findings of the physical examination combined with the medical history, the diagnosis of pneumonia, likely due to aspiration, is the most probable one in this case. This diagnosis in patients with advanced dementia and difficulties in swallowing carries a high mortality rate even with treatment. From Table 13.1, it is clear that this case is very high risk, with a predicted 14-day mortality of 75%, as all high-risk factors are present except for respiratory rate and pulse rate, which are close to the mean.

The family is in distress. Having an uncertain prognosis and seeing a loved one suffer are stressful. Identifying the diagnosis, unfolding the possible scenarios, and thereby marking the palliative phase is helpful in alleviating the uncertainty and thereby feelings of distress, even though the delivered message is somber. Discussing the possible treatment options should include not only curative approaches for the pneumonia but also options to treat symptoms only. Often family members have an (unspoken) fear of suffocation or starvation for their loved ones or have witnessed a troubled death before. Asking about concerns and experiences gives room to address implicit assumptions and align both family and the healthcare team to the optimal care plan.

TABLE 13.1. **Risk Factors for 14-Day Mortality**

Risk Factor for 14-Day Mortality	Present Case	PneuMonitor Study[1,2]
Male gender	Present	43%
Respiratory rate	33	Mean 25 (SD 8)
Respiratory difficulty	Present	56%
Heart rate	88	Mean 91 (SD 17)
Decreased alertness	Present	30%
Insufficient fluid intake	Present	51%
Dehydration	Present	30%
Eating dependency (independent, requires assistance, fully dependent)	Fully dependent	Independent 21%, requires assistance 36%, fully dependent 43%
Increase in eating dependency during the 2 weeks before diagnosis	Present	34%
Bowel incontinence	Present	62%
Cardiovascular history	Present	49%
14-day mortality		
with antibiotic treatment	Predicted 75%	14% overall in study population

See www.evidencio.com for algorithm.

ANTIBIOTICS OR NO ANTIBIOTICS

Mortality in a patient with a lower respiratory tract infection and advanced dementia is substantial despite antibiotics or hospital care. Antibiotic treatment, if given, may prolong life only for a few days or even with recovery for a few months. A helpful question about any treatment in this setting is whether treatment is prolonging living or prolonging the dying process. There is also uncertainty as to whether antibiotics play a significant role in the maintenance of comfort. Decisions about whether to prescribe or whether to hospitalize (an option frequently considered in the United

States) should take into consideration the risks and benefits of assessing and treating infections and the uncertainty regarding any significant benefits of treatment for patient comfort or prolonging life. These decisions should align with the goals and burden of care and treatment preferences as appropriate.

If treatment is considered, amoxicillin three times daily 500 mg (or in severe penicillin allergy doxycycline 200 mg on day 1 and then 100 mg/day thereafter, or clarithromycin twice daily 500 mg) represents a suitable treatment option, with a treatment duration of 5 days. Oral administration in this case may require syrup/liquid or orodispersible formulations due to dysphagia. An option to oral administration is intramuscular or subcutaneous ceftriaxone (1–2 g/day).

FOOD AND FLUIDS

Intake is problematic; swallowing dysfunction is already present, and the somnolent state of the patient is contributing to further risk of aspiration. Feeding tubes have not shown benefits in patients with advanced dementia in terms of preventing malnutrition, preventing complications, or prolonging life; this is mostly due to the fact that there is still the risk of aspiration with a feeding tube and the underlying cachexia is only partly caused by malnutrition. In terms of reducing symptom burden, tubes are often considered uncomfortable, both when being inserted and when in situ. Moreover, physical restraint might be needed to prevent the patient from pulling the tube out. Therefore, in our case, the use of a feeding tube for food intake is not considered a viable option.

Dehydration in this situation will most probably be of an isotonic nature resulting in a relative low symptom burden. Correlations between thirst sensations and volume depletion are, at most, modest. The most cumbersome symptom is a dry mouth, particularly in the presence of oral respiration, which can be treated with frequent oral cleaning and the application of artificial saliva gel. If artificial hydration is considered, via tube, subcutaneous boluses, or intravenously, it should be taken into account that hydration might prolong the dying process by several days, with an increased symptom burden due to increased sputum production. There are different attitudes and beliefs concerning artificial hydration therapy worldwide based on culture and medical education, and the evidence is not conclusive. However, experts agree that it is appropriate in the palliative phase not to start artificial rehydration. Comfort feeding by hand, if the patients shows a need for intake and exhibits an adequate swallowing reflex, would be an option. Consulting a speech and language therapist to assess the risks might be considered. Hand feeding by the family or otherwise oral cleaning and applying artificial saliva or applying fat to the lips to prevent hydration might reduce the sense of powerlessness in the family present at the bedside.

SYMPTOM OBSERVATION AND TREATMENT

Dying from pneumonia generally has a higher symptom burden than dying from other causes. Dyspnea, delirium and anxiety, pain, and general discomfort should be closely monitored so that palliative measures can be implemented in a timely and appropriate manner. Various symptom scales are available and should be considered for use by nursing staff, depending on their level of training.

Dyspnea

Dyspnea is the sensation of not getting enough breath. It can be classified in patients who cannot adequately communicate their symptom burden by use of, for instance, the Respiratory Distress Observation Scale (RDOS). Dyspnea is considered a symptom that involves a high burden of discomfort and should be treated where possible.

Nonpharmaceutical interventions are relevant and include a seated bed position and the use of a fan. The use of oxygen is debatable as the sensation of dyspnea is often not directly linked to the oxygen level; a trial of oxygen administration can be evaluated for effects on the level of dyspnea, taking into account the possible discomfort caused by the noise and the mouth-drying effect of the oxygen flow. Suction of mucus is not advisable as the intervention itself causes discomfort and its effect is short-lived. Further, the act of suction stimulates the production of more mucus.

The primary pharmaceutical intervention is the administration of morphine. Other opioids are being considered but so far have shown equivocal effects on dyspnea. As oral intake in this case is compromised, morphine can be applied subcutaneously, either continuously via a pump or as a bolus with injections via a subcutaneous entrance port. The starting dosage of morphine for dyspnea is much lower than the dosage indicated for pain. If only dyspnea is being treated, the starting dose should be ~0.5–1.0 mg/hour or 2.5 mg every 4 hours. An alternative to subcutaneous administration is the use of morphine concentrates of 20 mg/mL sublingually; as oral morphine has a potency of one-third of the parenteral route, the starting dose would generally be 5–10 mg sublingually every 1 hour as needed, with increases as needed until adequate symptom relief is obtained. Usually, the use of an opioid necessitates concomitant laxative use; however, in this palliative phase, with a short life expectancy and difficulties with oral intake, this is not appropriate.

Sometimes the use of bronchodilators such as inhaled salbutamol can reduce the symptom burden. Again, the discomfort of the use of a nebulizer should be evaluated against the achieved symptom relief.

Fever

Fever in itself is not a symptom that should be treated per se, unless it causes discomfort in the patient. A cool environment and thin cotton clothing and bedsheets may be sufficient. If not, antipyretics can be considered, which will also yield some pain reduction. However, in this case, this would require turning the patient in bed to administer via the rectal route.

Pain

Pain is an indirect effect of the respiratory infection. It is often caused by lengthy immobility in the same bed position and overall malaise. In nonresponsive patients such as ours, the use of a monitoring scale is strongly advised. There are several available; in this instance the Pain Assessment in Advanced Dementia (PAINAD) scale is applicable and sufficiently easy to use without training. Pain is often recognized rather late, and it might prove a challenge to distinguish it and/or anxiety from dyspnea. Nevertheless, it is advisable to immediately start using a pain scale when the diagnosis of pneumonia has been made, so as to detect pain promptly and not delay the use of appropriate pain medication.

Nonpharmaceutical interventions, which also serve as prevention measures, involving changing bed position on a regular basis and using appropriate bedding to prevent pressure ulcers. Pharmaceutically, opioids are the most logical choice, due to their effects on dyspnea, with a dosage also suitable to alleviate pain. The use of subcutaneous morphine is preferable over transdermal opioids as titration against symptom burden is easier and faster, which can reduce the time in discomfort.

Neuropsychiatric Symptoms

Neuropsychiatric symptoms should be expected, including anxiety due to dyspnea and restlessness with pain, but also delirium resulting in agitation and/or apathy. Patients with dementia have a much higher risk of developing delirium. Use of a Delirium Observation Screening (DOS) scale should be considered to monitor this. Pain, dyspnea, urine retention, or a full rectum or fecaloma should be treated. A trusted environment (the patient's own bedroom) with trusted faces (family and staff); short, calm, and friendly instructions and validations; and promoting a diurnal rhythm by opening curtains during daytime and promoting adequate rest at night are helpful.

Delirium can be treated with antipsychotic medication, although there is increasing research that its effect might be limited or even negative. Haloperidol is in general the agent of choice, but in Parkinson's disease dementia or Lewy body dementia it is contraindicated. The most commonly used antipsychotics would be quetiapine or clozapine. However, oral administration is difficult in our case, which would suggest either clozapine 12.5 mg orally or in buccal form or olanzapine 5 mg orally, give intramuscularly or via orodispersible tablets as an alternative for quetiapine. The use of a benzodiazepine, such as lorazepam or midazolam, should also be considered.

MEDICATION REVIEW

The patient's medications should be reviewed. In our case the enalapril and acetylsalicylic acid can be stopped, as the indications for preventive measures are no longer applicable. Macrogol and acetaminophen are still indicated, macrogol to prevent obstipation associated with opioid use and acetaminophen to combat pain and fever. Both should be stopped due to compromised oral intake; acetaminophen might be switched to rectal administration. Newly added medications will be subcutaneous or oral morphine, artificial saliva, possible salbutamol and oxygen, and clonazepam and/or midazolam if delirium develops.

FAMILY GUIDANCE

In this phase, daily conversations with the family are recommended. The process will often take anywhere from a couple of days to a week, and these days can prove very long for the next of kin. Reiteration of the care plan, unfolding of possible scenarios, advising possible actions they might perform (mouth care, possible comfort feeding, creating a calm and reassuring environment, familiar music in the background, hand touch) and, in a later stage, predicting Cheyne–Stokes breathing patterns or explaining death rattle in advance all contribute toward relieving anxiety in the family. Moreover, it shows them that their loved one is still receiving optimal appropriate medical care, even though cure is no longer the aim.

KEY POINTS TO REMEMBER

- Pneumonia in advanced dementia carries a high mortality rate but also a high symptom burden. The use of observation scales is highly recommended to detect possible symptoms promptly.
- Changes in the severity of symptoms or the onset of symptoms should be quickly acted upon.
- Nonpharmaceutical interventions should not be overlooked. They can bring relief and also help family members feel less powerless.
- The family requires daily support. This is a time for reiterating the care plan and the scenario unfolding as well as for carefully listening to their (often implicit) concerns.

Further Reading

Arcand M. End-of-life issues in advanced dementia, part 2: management of poor nutritional intake, dehydration, and pneumonia. *Can Fam Physician.* 2015;61:337–341.

Campbell ML, Templin TN, Walch J. A respiratory distress observation scale for patients unable to self-report dyspnea. *J Palliat Med.* 2010;13(3):285–290.

Campbell ML, Kero KK, Templin TN. Mild, moderate, and severe intensity cut-points for the Respiratory Distress Observation Scale. *Heart Lung*. 2017;46(1):14–17.

Gavinski K, Carnahan R, Weckmann M. Validation of the delirium observation screening scale in a hospitalized older population. *J Hosp Med*. 2016;11(7):494–497.

Mitchell SL. Care of patients with advanced dementia. July 2019, UpToDate.

van der Maaden T, de Vet HC, Achterberg WP, et al. Improving comfort in people with dementia and pneumonia: a cluster randomized trial. *BMC Med*. 2016;14:116.

van der Steen JT, Lane P, Kowall NW, et al. Antibiotics and mortality in patients with lower respiratory infection and advanced dementia. *J Am Med Dir Assoc*. 2012;13(2):156–161.

van der Steen JT, Radbruch L, Hertogh CM, et al. White paper defining optimal palliative care in older people with dementia: a Delphi study and recommendations from the European Association for Palliative Care. *Palliat Med*. 2014;28(3):197–209.

Volicer L. Chapter 14.1, Palliative medicine in dementia. In: *Oxford Textbook of Palliative Management*, 4th ed. Oxford University Press; 2010:1375–1385.

Warden V, Hurley AC, Volicer L. Development and psychometric evaluation of the Pain Assessment in Advanced Dementia (PAINAD) scale. *J Am Med Dir Assoc*. 2003;4(1):9–15.

References

1. Rauh SP, Heymans MW, van der Maaden T, et al. Predicting mortality in nursing home residents with dementia and pneumonia treated with antibiotics: validation of a prediction model in a more recent population. *J Gerontol A*. 2019;74(12):1922–1928.

2. van der Maaden T, van der Steen JT, de Vet HC, et al. Prospective observations of discomfort, pain, and dyspnea in nursing home residents with dementia and pneumonia. *J Am Med Dir Assoc*. 2016;17:128–135.

14 Last Days with Chronic Obstructive Pulmonary Disease

Margaret L. Campbell

The hospice nurse makes an initial home visit to Maxwell and his wife, Althea. Maxwell, 78 years old, has end-stage chronic obstructive pulmonary disease (COPD) and was discharged from the hospital yesterday, where he had a long stay, including intensive care.

The nurse notes signs of respiratory distress. Maxwell is sitting forward in a recliner with his elbows on his knees; wheezing is audible. She estimates his respiratory rate at 32. Supplemental oxygen is flowing at 4 L/minute. Meter-dose inhalers (MDIs) are on a nearby table. Maxwell is very thin. Lung sounds are distant. He can speak only one or two words between breaths.

Althea reports that she has had difficulty helping him walk from the recliner to the bathroom, which is down the hall; he pauses often for breath and is exhausted after using the bathroom and must rest on the toilet until he can make the arduous trip back to the recliner.

What do I do now?

Patients approaching the end of life will benefit from hospice care; patients are eligible if a prescribing clinician estimates that life expectancy is 6 months or less. The eligibility criteria for hospice enrollment when the diagnosis is COPD are as follows:

- Recent visits to the emergency department or hospitalization for pulmonary infections or respiratory failure
- Dyspnea or tightness in the chest (FEV$_1$ <30% of predicted)
- Identification of specific structural/functional impairments
- Relevant activity limitations
- Changes in appetite and unintentional progressive weight loss
- Impaired sleep functions
- Decline in general physical endurance
- Impaired mobility
- Requires oxygen some of the time or all of the time
- May require breathing treatments or use of inhalers
- May have difficulty eating or carrying on conversations without becoming short of breath

Maxwell meets all these eligibility criteria. His treatment goals are dyspnea comfort-focused. Several activities of daily living must be modified to accommodate his declining function as well as medications and routes of delivery.

NUTRITION

Appetite dwindles in all late-stage disease. Persons with advanced COPD may not eat enough secondary to dyspnea; it is difficulty to chew and swallow while tachypneic. Soft, easy-to-swallow foods that require little or no chewing such as soups, oatmeal, or scrambled eggs are recommended. Liquid nutrition supplements may also be palatable and easy to swallow.

PACING ACTIVITY

Balancing activity with rest is an important consideration. Even the most basic activities of daily living can exacerbate dyspnea in the end stages of COPD. Eating breakfast, bathing, and dressing may need to be staggered over hours rather than minutes. Rearranging furniture to afford places to sit and rest when the patient moves from one room to another can be tried. As mobility declines, the patient may always be in a single room with meals brought to the bed or chair. A wheelchair may be necessary.

TOILETING

Walking to and from the bathroom may be too strenuous for a person with COPD who has continuous dyspnea. A wheelchair may or may not be accessible depending on the size of the bathroom. Durable medical equipment is covered by insurance under the hospice benefit; a commode can be placed near the bed or chair, allowing for fewer steps. The family caregiver can be taught how to assist the patient to stand, pivot, and sit.

POSITIONING

Patients with COPD benefit most from an upright position with the arms supported. This increases the vital capacity and may increase oxygen and carbon dioxide exchange. A recliner is ideal because it has arm supports and can be adjusted to a patient-specific angle for sleep. A hospital bed may also be useful to provide upright positioning. In the case of a dyspnea exacerbation, COPD patients may be assisted by leaning forward and resting their elbows on their knees or thighs. This tripod position resembles what runners do when they reach a breathing capacity limit.

SUPPLEMENTAL OXYGEN

There are two central drivers for breathing, hypercarbia and hypoxemia. Because COPD patients spend their lives chronically hypercarbic, the central nervous system no longer responds to that stimulus, and their only trigger for breathing is the level of oxygen (or lack thereof) in their blood. Supplemental O_2 may remove a COPD patient's hypoxemic respiratory drive, causing hypoventilation with resultant hypercarbia, apnea, and ultimate respiratory failure. Thus, caution must be given to increasing supplemental oxygen when the patient is chronically hypercarbic and hypoxemic.

Increasing the flow of air to the face may reduce dyspnea. Opening a window near the patient's bed or chair, weather permitting, may be helpful. A handheld or tabletop fan directed at the face can be effective.[1]

MEDICATIONS

Long-acting bronchodilators and anticholinergics every 12 hours by MDI are the mainstay of COPD treatment, along with short-acting agents as needed for breakthrough dyspnea. In their last days, patients may not be able to use the MDI effectively. Changing to an aerosol route is indicated; the family caregiver can be taught by the hospice staff how to measure and deliver the medication. These medications should be continued until the patient becomes unconscious.

Immediate-release oral morphine is an effective treatment for dyspnea.[2] Morphine alters central perception of hypercarbia and hypoxemia. For the opioid-naïve patient, an initial dose of 5 mg may be sufficient. This may be administered every 4 hours around the clock with an as-needed dose every 1 hour. Constipation is the most common adverse effect; thus, a bowel regimen is indicated when initiating morphine.

Continuous dyspnea contributes to the development of anxiety in some patients. Benzodiazepines may be effective to treat anxiety and moderate sleep disorders but do not have a primary effect on reducing dyspnea.[3] These agents should be used cautiously as the adverse events of sedation and risk of falls need to be considered.

TRAJECTORY OF DYSPNEA AT THE END OF LIFE

Patients with chronic dyspnea may experience an escalation during the last days secondary to progressive respiratory failure and weakening of chest muscles. In two studies dyspnea increased in the last week of life.[4,5] The last week of life can be predicted by reliance on the Palliative Performance Scale; a score of 10 indicates the last week.[6,7] Close attention to patient report or signs of respiratory distress by the hospice clinicians and the family caregiver will ensure that appropriate techniques to relieve distress are implemented.

Mitchell was displaying signs of and reporting shortness of breath. Althea indicated that Mitchell struggled to walk anywhere in their home.

They reported that he was comfortable in the recliner since he could raise or lower the head or feet to accommodate his changing comfort. The nurse ordered a commode that could be placed next to the chair, obviating the need to walk to the bathroom. The chair was near a window and weather permitted keeping it open to permit airflow. Supplemental oxygen was maintained at 4 L/min. The nurse asked Mitchell to demonstrate MDI use and she noted his shaking hands and difficulty with administration, so the MDIs were converted to aerosol treatments. Mitchell had received small doses of morphine while hospitalized, which imparted relief; a prescription for immediate-release oral morphine 5 mg every 4 hours, with 5 mg every 1 hour as needed, was sent to the pharmacy. A bowel regimen with senna 2 tablets at bedtime was also prescribed.

The nurse recognized that Mitchell was in the last 1–2 weeks of life and planned house calls twice weekly with home health aides three times weekly to assist with bathing, dressing, and volunteer time so Althea could occasionally get out of the house.

KEY POINTS TO REMEMBER

- Dyspnea is often continuous for patients with advanced COPD and escalates near death.
- Bronchodilators may need to be administered as aerosol treatments instead of MDIs.
- Immediate-release morphine in a concentrated formulation can be administered in the buccal space to trickle into the pharynx and be swallowed when consciousness is waning.

References
1. Luckett T, Phillips J, Johnson MJ, et al. Contributions of a hand-held fan to self-management of chronic breathlessness. *Eur Respir J*. 2017;50(2):1700262.
2. Jennings AL, Davies AN, Higgins JP, Gibbs JS, Broadley KE. A systematic review of the use of opioids in the management of dyspnoea. *Thorax*. 2002;57(11):939–944.
3. Simon ST, Higginson IJ, Booth S, Harding R, Weingartner V, Bausewein C. Benzodiazepines for the relief of breathlessness in advanced malignant and non-malignant diseases in adults. *Cochrane Database Syst Rev*. 2016;10:CD007354.

4. Campbell ML, Kiernan JM, Strandmark J, Yarandi HN. Trajectory of dyspnea and respiratory distress among patients in the last month of life. *J Palliat Med.* 2018;21(2):194–199.

5. Currow DC, Smith J, Davidson PM, Newton PJ, Agar MR, Abernethy AP. Do the trajectories of dyspnea differ in prevalence and intensity by diagnosis at the end of life? A consecutive cohort study. *J Pain Symptom Manage.* 2010;39(4):680–690.

6. Harrold J, Rickerson E, Carroll JT, et al. Is the Palliative Performance Scale a useful predictor of mortality in a heterogeneous hospice population? *J Palliat Med.* 2005;8(3):503–509.

7. Weng L-C, Huang H-L, Wilkie D, et al. Predicting survival with the Palliative Performance Scale in a minority-serving hospice and palliative care program. *J Pain Symptom Manage.* 2009;37:642–648.

15 Withdrawal of Invasive Mechanical Ventilation

Margaret L. Campbell

Estelle, a 73-year-old woman, presented to the emergency department with difficulty breathing secondary to aspiration pneumonia, associated with advanced-stage dementia. She required invasive mechanical ventilation (MV), and admission to the medical intensive care unit (MICU). A decision was made to withdraw mechanical ventilation and allow a natural death.

On physical examination she was responsive to voice and touch but did not follow commands. She was restless and attempted to pull on her catheters and endotracheal tube despite wrist restraints. Heart rate was 120 and respiratory rate was 28. She had an oral endotracheal tube. Ventilator settings were the Assist Control mode with a set rate of 14, tidal volume (Vt) 300 cc, and fraction of inspired oxygen (FiO_2) at 0.40, with positive-pressure end-expiratory pressure (PEEP) at 5 cm. Her peripheral oxygen saturation (SpO_2) ranged from 93% to 98%.

Assurances were made to the family that Estelle's respiratory comfort would be a priority during ventilator withdrawal.

What do I do now?

For decades, MV has been used to support breathing in patients experiencing acute or chronic respiratory failure. MV is of benefit when the patient, for a number of reasons, cannot maintain normal ventilation as evidenced by increasing carbon dioxide and respiratory acidosis. Both invasive and noninvasive MV modalities are employed. Invasive MV is applied using an artificial airway such as an endotracheal tube or tracheostomy. Noninvasive MV is applied over the nose or nose and mouth via a tight-fitting face mask. Examples of noninvasive MV include continuous positive airway pressure (CPAP) or bilevel positive airway pressure (BiPAP).

Invasive MV is employed after cardiopulmonary arrest, during general anesthesia, to treat respiratory failure that is not responsive to noninvasive ventilation, or for patients who are ventilator-dependent. Endotracheal intubation is used for periods of less than 2 weeks of ventilation; continued ventilation after 2 weeks is supported by tracheostomy.

Patients often experience discomfort during MV. Endotracheal intubation causes gagging, coughing, and drooling and leaves the patient unable to verbalize because the tube passes through the vocal cords. In many cases of endotracheal intubation, the patient requires mechanical restraints or sedation to maintain the integrity of the life-saving treatment and to ensure ventilator synchrony.

Ventilator withdrawal is considered as a treatment option when the treatment is more burdensome than beneficial, such as when patients have a terminal illness or are unconscious or when patients make an informed, capable decision to cease treatment because their quality of life is poor. Ventilator withdrawal is conducted to allow a natural death free of tubes and machines.

Patients are ventilated because of respiratory failure and an inability to exchange respiratory gases without mechanical support; they are at high risk for developing dyspnea and post-extubation stridor. Dyspnea arises from increased inspiratory effort, hypercarbia, and/or hypoxemia. Prevention and alleviation of dyspnea or respiratory distress becomes the focus of care. Some patients, if awake, may experience fear or anxiety before or during ventilator withdrawal, which will require attention if present. Adult patients may experience barotrauma to the trachea from the pressure in the cuff, leading to laryngeal edema or spasm after extubation with development of post-extubation stridor.

ADVANCE PREPARATION

The Centers for Medicare and Medicaid Services (CMMS) has enacted guidelines for consistent processes around organ donation. Hospital staff must notify their state Organ Procurement Organization (OPO) when decisions about ventilator withdrawal are being considered. The OPO will collaborate with the hospital staff to identify whether the patient is a candidate for donation after cardiac death and to seek consent from the next of kin. This evaluation by the OPO must be completed before ventilation is withdrawn.[1]

The timing of the withdrawal process is generally negotiated with the patient's family and the healthcare team. This timing will depend on which team members will be present, including support personnel, such as a chaplain. The time needs to be communicated to all clinical team members, and ideally the assigned nurse should have a reduced assignment to be able to spend 1:1 time with the patient and family.

Not all family members want to be present at the bedside during withdrawal. Another room nearby can be arranged with adequate seating, tissues, and water. Religious observances or family-specific rituals need to be accommodated and completed before beginning the withdrawal process. Patient and/or family questions about what to expect can be addressed before beginning the process.

Neuromuscular blocking agents (NMBAs), such as pancuronium or vecuronium, are being used with less frequency in the ICU. When in use, it is impossible to assess the patient's comfort. Thus, the NMBA should be discontinued with evidence of patient neuromuscular recovery before ventilator withdrawal is undertaken. In some cases, the duration of action of these agents is prolonged, such as when the patient has liver or renal failure and impaired clearance. Therefore, although controversial, withdrawal can proceed with careful attention to ensuring patient comfort if an unacceptable delay in withdrawing MV occurs because of protracted effects of NMBA.

MEASURING DISTRESS

Dyspnea, also known as breathlessness, is a nociceptive phenomenon defined as "a subjective experience of breathing discomfort that consists of qualitatively distinct sensations that vary in intensity. The experience derives from interactions among multiple physiological, psychological, social and environmental factors, and may induce secondary physiological and behavioral responses."[2] Dyspnea can be perceived and verified only by the person experiencing it. Many patients who are undergoing ventilator withdrawal are cognitively impaired or unconscious as a result of underlying neurological lesions or hemodynamic, metabolic, or respiratory dysfunction. Respiratory distress is an observable (behavioral) corollary to dyspnea; the physical and emotional suffering that results from the experience of asphyxiation is characterized by behaviors that can be observed and measured.[3]

Most patients undergoing ventilator withdrawal will be unable to provide a self-report about any dyspnea experienced, particularly patients who are unconscious or severely cognitively impaired. Attempts to elicit a self-report should be made if the patient is conscious. Skill is required to detect nuances of behaviors, particularly when the patient is unable to validate the clinician's assessment. Initiation and escalation of sedatives and opioids should be guided by patient behaviors.

The Respiratory Distress Observation Scale (RDOS) is suitable for assessing the adult patient during the withdrawal of mechanical ventilation; reliability, validity, and intensity cut-points have been established.[3-5] This eight-variable categorical scale is the only known tool for assessing respiratory distress when the patient cannot self-report dyspnea, which typifies most patients undergoing ventilator withdrawal. Each variable is scored from 0 to 2 points and the points are summed. Scores range from 0 to 16: 0–2 = no distress, 3 = mild distress, 4–6 moderate distress, and 7 or higher = severe distress (Table 15.1). Brain-dead patients will not show distress, cough, gag, or breathe during or following ventilator withdrawal, and sedation or analgesia is not indicated.

PREMEDICATION FOR ANTICIPATED DISTRESS

As is the standard with pain management, opioids should be initiated at signs of distress, and the advice to "start low and titrate slowly" is sage. For the opioid-naïve adult an initial intravenous bolus of 3–5 mg morphine is recommended. Anticipatory premedication is a sound practice if distress is already evident and if distress can be anticipated. There is no justification

TABLE 15.1. **Respiratory Distress Observation Scale**

Variable	0 points	1 point	2 points	Total
Heart rate per minute	<90 beats	91–109 beats	≥110 beats	
Respiratory rate per minute	≤18 breaths	19–30 breaths	>30 breaths	
Restlessness: non-purposeful movements	None	Occasional, slight movements	Frequent movements	
Accessory muscle use: rise in clavicle during inspiration	None	Slight rise	Pronounced rise	
Paradoxical breathing: abdomen moves in on inspiration	None		Present	
Grunting at end-expiration: guttural sound	None		Present	
Nasal flaring: involuntary movement of nares	None		Present	
Look of fear	None		Eyes wide open, facial muscles tense, brow furrowed, mouth open	
Total				

Margaret L. Campbell, PhD, RN.

for medicating a brain-dead patient, and one could argue that the patient in coma with only minimal brainstem function is also unlikely to experience distress. Doses that correspond to customary dosing for the treatment of dyspnea should guide dosing during ventilator withdrawal.

Documentation of the signs of distress or the RDOS score and the rationale for dose escalation is important to ensure continuity across professional caregivers and to prevent overmedication and the appearance of hastening death. At the conclusion of the process a continuous infusion may be initiated to maintain patient comfort; an infusion rate equivalent to 50% of the total amount of bolus medication is recommended. Thus, if the patient received three boluses of morphine at 4 mg (12 mg), the infusion would start at a rate of 6 mg/hr.

WEANING METHOD

Terminal extubation is characterized by ceasing ventilatory support and removing the endotracheal tube in one step. *Terminal weaning* is a process of stepwise, gradual reductions in oxygen and ventilation, terminating with placement of a T-piece or with extubation. Patients undergoing terminal extubation experienced more distress than patients with terminal weaning.[6–7] Terminal extubation poses an abrupt change from supported ventilation to spontaneous ventilation in a fragile patient, likely contributing to the distress observed in these studies.

Rapid terminal weaning may afford the clinician with the most control because it allows for careful, sequential adjustments to the ventilator with precise titration of medications to ensure patient comfort[5] (Table 15.2). Continuous patient monitoring with readily accessible intravenous opioids will afford the patient with comfort regardless of the method employed.

EXTUBATION CONSIDERATIONS

Patients who are ventilator-dependent for 14 days or more are generally ventilated through a tracheostomy tube. After ventilator withdrawal a tracheostomy collar with humidified room air or low-flow oxygen can be placed. Patients experiencing acute respiratory failure are ventilated through a nasal or oral endotracheal tube. Adult tubes have a cuff to maintain tube placement and occlude the trachea to prevent air leakage and loss of tidal volume.

Removal of the endotracheal tube should be performed whenever possible because of patient comfort and the aesthetic appearance of the patient. However, in some cases airway compromise can be anticipated, such

TABLE 15.2. **Sample Rapid Wean**

Process	Steps	Rationale
Planning	Cuff-leak testing	Affords prediction of post-extubation stridor
Premedication: Patients able to experience distress (e.g. RASS +3 to –3)	Morphine 4 mg IV bolus	Morphine is effective for treating dyspnea. Comatose patients may not need premedication but should be monitored for development of distress.
Weaning	1. Turn off PEEP. 2. Wean FiO$_2$ by 0.2 every 1–2 minutes if no distress until FiO$_2$ = 0.21 (room air). 3. Change ventilator mode to SIMV at a rate of 10 with PSV at 5 cm. 4. Reduce SIMV rate by 2 breaths every 1–2 minutes if no distress until SIMV rate = 4. 5. Change ventilator mode to CPAP 0, PSV 5 cm. 6. Turn off ventilator and remove from patient. 7. Extubate if cuff leak test passed.	Stepwise weaning affords an opportunity to pause the process when distress develops. Patients are given the opportunity to "adjust" to each change rather than rapidly being changed from full ventilation to complete spontaneous breathing.
Assess distress	Measure RDOS at baseline and after every ventilator change.	Patients may develop respiratory distress anywhere along the trajectory from fully supported ventilation to spontaneous breathing.
Treat distress	Morphine 4 mg IV bolus whenever RDOS is ≥4.	RDOS 0–2 = no distress, 3 = mild distress.

(continued)

TABLE 15.2. **Continued**

Process	Steps	Rationale
Maintain comfort	Morphine infusion if patient needed medication during withdrawal and if predicted survival is more than minutes. Calculate the total morphine given during withdrawal as bolus doses. Begin infusion at a rate = 50% of total bolus doses.	Patients may survive longer than minutes and can be triaged to a non-ICU bed. Nurse–patient ratios on non-ICU units do not afford frequent IV bolus dosing.
	Titrate to maintain RDOS ≤ 3.	
Treat stridor	Racemic epinephrine in 3 cc normal saline as an aerosol treatment. May need to be repeated ×1.	Opioids and benzodiazepines will not treat airway obstruction.

CPAP = continuous positive airway pressure, IV = intravenous, FiO_2 = fraction of inspired air, PEEP = positive end-expiratory pressure, RASS = Richmond Agitation Severity Scale, RDOS = Respiratory Distress Observation Scale, SIMV = synchronized intermittent mandatory ventilation.

as when the patient has a swollen, protuberant tongue or has pulmonary hemorrhage. Medication with dexamethasone may reduce airway edema, permitting extubation when patients are at high risk for post-extubation laryngeal edema, but dosing would need to start 12 hours before withdrawal if the timing permits. Aerosolized racemic epinephrine is a useful intervention to reduce stridor after extubation. Family counseling about the usual noises that can be expected and that cause no distress should be done prior to extubation.

OXYGEN

A growing body of evidence suggests that oxygen is a useful palliative intervention to treat dyspnea when the patient is experiencing distress and is hypoxemic but offers no benefit when the patient has normal oxygenation. Further, when patients are near death and in no distress, oxygen is not necessary.[8] Thus, the patient can be cared for without oxygen following ventilator withdrawal unless there are signs of respiratory distress and hypoxemia. A nasal cannula is better tolerated than a face mask if oxygen is initiated.

DURATION OF SURVIVAL

Triage considerations after ventilator withdrawal may be guided by estimates of duration of survival. As expected, patients with the highest illness severity will die more quickly, particularly if they are also dependent on vasopressors or high levels of oxygen.

SUMMARY

Withdrawal of mechanical ventilation is a procedure that occurs with relative frequency. The benefits of this therapy, when initiated, is to replace failing lungs, extend life, and improve quality of life by relieving dyspnea associated with respiratory failure. When the burdens exceed the benefits, or when the patient is near death or unresponsive, decisions may be made to cease this therapy. Measures to palliate anticipated distress must be applied. A peaceful death after cessation of mechanical ventilation can be provided.

Returning to our case, Estelle was not able to respond to commands but did withdraw from painful stimuli. Thus, it was presumed that she could experience distress. Further, she was ventilator-dependent and at high risk for developing respiratory distress during spontaneous breathing. For these reasons she was premedicated with morphine 4 mg and 1 mg of lorazepam in an intravenous bolus.

A rapid terminal weaning was undertaken in which oxygen and ventilation were reduced in stepwise fashion until Estelle was breathing spontaneously. During the stepwise weaning she was monitored with the RDOS. At each step she was re-medicated with morphine 4 mg if the RDOS score indicated the presence of respiratory distress. She required two bolus doses of morphine during the weaning process; total morphine administered was 12 mg.

The ventilator was turned off. A continuous morphine infusion at 6 mg/hr was initiated to maintain respiratory comfort. Estelle died 4 hours after ventilator withdrawal.

References

1. Centers for Medicare and Medicaid Services. Organ Procurement Organization (OPO) Conditions for Coverage Final Rule: Revisions to Outcome Measures for OPOs CMS-3380-F. 2020. https://www.cms.gov/newsroom/fact-sheets/organ-proc urement-organization-opo-conditions-coverage-final-rule-revisions-outcome-measures-opos

2. Parshall MB, Schwartzstein RM, Adams L, et al. An official American Thoracic Society statement: update on the mechanisms, assessment, and management of dyspnea. *Am J Respir Crit Care Med.* 2012;185(4):435–452.

3. Campbell ML, Templin T, Walch J. A Respiratory Distress Observation Scale for patients unable to self-report dyspnea. *J Palliat Med.* 2010;13(3):285–290.

4. Campbell ML, Kero KK, Templin TN. Mild, moderate, and severe intensity cut-points for the Respiratory Distress Observation Scale. *Heart Lung.* 2017;46(1):14–17.

5. Campbell ML, Templin TN. Intensity cut-points for the Respiratory Distress Observation Scale. *Palliat Med.* 2015;29(5):436–442.

6. Campbell ML, Yarandi HN, Mendez M. A two-group trial of a terminal ventilator withdrawal algorithm: pilot testing. *J Palliat Med.* 2015;18(9):781–785.

7. Robert R, Le Gouge A, Kentish-Barnes N, et al. Terminal weaning or immediate extubation for withdrawing mechanical ventilation in critically ill patients (the ARREVE observational study). *Intensive Care Med.* 2017;43(12):1793–1807.

8. Campbell ML, Yarandi H, Dove-Medows E. Oxygen is nonbeneficial for most patients who are near death. *J Pain Symptom Manage.* 2013;45(3):517–523.

16 Palliative Sedation for Intractable Dyspnea

Patricia Bramati and Eduardo Bruera

The patient is a 76-year-old male diagnosed with non-small cell lung cancer 5 years ago for which he underwent a right upper lobectomy. The patient presents today with shortness of breath that has developed over the last few months. Initially it was only present with moderate effort but it has progressed to be at rest, and to the point that he is unable to talk in full sentences. The chest x-ray showed a reticulonodular pattern, with thickening of the interlobular septa suggestive of lymphangitis carcinomatosis and lesions in the ribs compatible with bone metastasis. The patient was started on diuretics, antibiotics, steroids, inhalers, and high-flow oxygen via nasal cannula. His shortness of breath did not improve, and his oxygen saturation was 83%. Opioids and corticosteroids were titrated to dose-limiting toxicity but the patient remained severely breathless. After discussing goals of care, the patient and family asked for a do-not-resuscitate order and to stop the suffering.

What do I do now?

atitles with advanced cancer develop a number of devastating physical and psychosocial symptoms. Breathlessness is very common in patients in palliative care and tends to increase over the course of advanced illnesses such as cancer, congestive heart failure, chronic pulmonary obstructive disease, and pulmonary fibrosis. It is one of the most common and most feared symptoms among cancer patients, occurring in ~20–40% at the time of diagnosis of advanced disease and up to 70% in the last 6 weeks of life.

Dyspnea is frequently multicausal in patients with advanced cancer. The main contributors can usually be determined in most patients by obtaining an adequate history, a physical examination, a chest-x-ray, and a blood workup. It is extremely important to identify treatable conditions (Table 16.1), but when the cause is irreversible or refractory, symptomatic relief of the shortness of breath becomes the priority. A combined approach using pharmacological treatment (opioids, bronchodilators, and corticosteroids) and nonpharmacological treatment (cooling the face, opening windows, using a small fan, adequate positioning, respiratory training, counseling) is frequently necessary to achieve symptomatic relief. Unfortunately, a significant proportion of patients develop refractory symptoms before death, and sedation, sometimes to unresponsiveness, becomes the only effective means of relieving suffering.

PALLIATIVE SEDATION

Palliative sedation, defined by the American Academy of Hospice and Palliative Medicine as the intentional lowering of awareness toward, and including, unconsciousness for patients with severe and refractory symptoms, is an ethically and legally well-accepted intervention. This definition, as others, implies symptom refractoriness and proportionality, and makes no distinction between continuous and intermittent, and light and deep sedation. The most common situations in which palliative sedation is used are terminal agitated delirium, refractory shortness of breath, and intractable pain.

For sedation to be indicated, symptoms must be refractory, meaning resistant to the treatment and not merely difficult to manage. As an example of the latter, treatments might be available but might take too long to be

TABLE 16.1. **Reversible Causes of Dyspnea in Cancer Patients and Treatment**

Direct effect of the tumor

Pleural effusion	Thoracentesis/drain
Pericardial effusion	Pericardiocentesis/drain/window
Superior cava syndrome	Stenting
Atelectasis	Chest percussion/bronchoscopy
Tracheal obstruction	Stenting

Effect of therapies

Radiation pneumonitis	Corticosteroids

Unrelated to tumor or cancer treatment

Anemia	Transfusion
Ascites	Paracentesis/drain
Chronic obstructive pulmonary disease	Corticosteroids/inhalers
Asthma	Corticosteroids/inhalers
Pulmonary emboli	Anticoagulation/embolectomy
Pneumothorax	Drain
Heart failure	Diuretics

Adapted from reference 4.

implemented, or the physician in charge might be uncomfortable using it. Additionally, controlling a symptom depends not only on its severity but also on the patient's perception.

The idea of proportionality means that palliative sedation should be administered in an "in crescendo" manner. Mild intermittent sedation should be considered first, and the level should be titrated according to the patient's level of awareness and symptom control. Even transient sedation, also known as respite sedation, may be attempted. In certain catastrophic situations, however, such as massive hemorrhage, asphyxiation, severe terminal dyspnea, or overwhelming pain crisis, the slow "in crescendo" approach might not be feasible, and continuous deep sedation might be required from the start.

The principle of double effect provides ethical guidance for decisions when all possible actions might result in a bad outcome. The first known example of double-effect reasoning is in Thomas Aquinas's (1225–1274) treatment of homicidal self-defense in his work *Summa Theologica*. This principle states that an action with two or more possible effects, including at least a "good" and at least a "bad" one, is morally permissible if four provisions are met: the action must not be immoral in itself; the action must be undertaken with the intention of achieving only the good effect (possible bad effects must be foreseen but not intended); the action must not achieve the good effect by means of a bad effect; and the action must be undertaken for a proportionally grave reason.

Some authors have criticized the doctrine's reliance on the intention of the physician because the intention can be complex, ambiguous, and often contradictory, while others consider that the loss of consciousness is not simply unintended but is in fact the means by which symptoms become controlled. In the case of palliative sedation, relieving the suffering is the intended good effect. Potential bad effects include respiratory depression, hypotension, and hastening death, which are foreseen but not intended. Palliative sedation is not immoral as long as the patient or surrogate requests this intervention, accepts the risks and benefits, and consents to it with the understanding that any other intervention has been unsuccessfully attempted.

When considering the use of palliative sedation, it is vital to be aware of each country's customs and laws about end-of-life issues. Great differences exist among nations and even among states in a single country. As an example, while in some cultures palliative sedation is unthinkable, France has recently passed a law giving patients the right to ask to avoid suffering and not to suffer unreasonable delays, recommending deep and continuous sedation until death in cases of intractable or unbearable pain if death is expected within the next few hours or days.

One of the most controversial aspects of this practice is the potential for shortening life. Two systematic reviews (Maltoni in 2012[1] and a Cochrane systematic review in 2015[2]) showed evidence that palliative sedation did not hasten death. However, these findings need to be considered with caution because most of the studies included in these systematic reviews were retrospective and a clear distinction was not always made between the primary intended sedation and secondary sedation, or between light and deep, intermittent and continuous, progressive (proportionate) and precipitous (sudden) sedation.

The medications used to achieve palliative sedation include benzodiazepines, chlorpromazine, barbiturates (phenobarbital or pentobarbital), and the anesthetics propofol and dexmedetomidine (Box 16.1). The most widely used medication is midazolam because of its rapid onset and short half-life and because it can be given intravenously or subcutaneously. Midazolam has sedative–hypnotic, anxiolytic, muscle relaxant, and anticonvulsant effects. The availability of a reversal agent, flumazenil, is a great advantage.

In our institution the use of midazolam for palliative sedation was initially limited to the intensive care unit. In the palliative care unit, chlorpromazine and/or lorazepam were used to control refractory symptoms. Later on, after the input of multiple hospital committees, including the ethics committee, the anesthesia service, and the medical practice committee, midazolam and propofol were approved for use in the palliative care unit.

The decision to pursue palliative sedation involves the participation of the patient (or a surrogate if the patient is unable), the primary team, the palliative team, and on occasions the ethics service. Once the decision is made to pursue palliative sedation, informed consent is obtained and

---

BOX 16.1. **Common Medications Used for Palliative Sedation and Starting Dose**

- Midazolam, 0.5–1.0 mg/hour. Rapid onset, short-acting, can be used IV or SC.
- Chlorpromazine, 12.5–25 mg IV/IM q 4–12 hours. Antipsychotic; can be used orally, IV, IM, rectally.
- Phenobarbital, 1–3 mg/kg IV or SC loading dose followed by 0.5 mg/kg/hour infusion.
- Propofol, 0.5 mg/kg/hour. Rapid onset; watch for hypotension and respiratory depression. Vial and any unused drug needs to be discarded after 12 hours.
- Dexmedetomidine, 0.1–0.4 mg/kg/hour. Watch for hypotension and bradycardia.

IM = intramuscularly, IV = intravenously, SC = subcutaneously.

documented in the medical record, the patient is moved to the palliative care unit, and a continuous infusion of midazolam (propofol is rarely used) is started. A single nurse is assigned to the patient during the initial 24 hours, and vital signs are monitored regularly. Patients continue to receive all symptom-control measures as appropriate. Per policy, the smallest effective dose of midazolam (or propofol) to control symptoms is used, and the need to continue palliative sedation is reassessed daily by the palliative care specialist. Monitoring the sedation is done clinically with the Richmond Agitation–Sedation Scale (RASS), a medical scale used to measure the patient's agitation or sedation level (Table 16.2); some authorities have suggested using bispectral index (BIS) monitoring. Attempts to lighten the sedation are considered if symptoms are controlled.

The decision of whether to continue hydration and artificial nutrition is independent from the decision to use palliative sedation and should be based on the patient's values, wishes, and medical condition. This decision should be addressed before the initiation of palliative sedation. If hydration is used, it should be frequently reviewed and stopped if it is causing harm.

In our palliative care unit, there were 1,207 admissions in 2004 and 2005.[3] Of these patients, 186 (15%) received palliative sedation. The median age of patients who received palliative sedation was 58, and 57% were male. The most common indications for palliative sedation were delirium (82%) and dyspnea (6%). Midazolam was used in 18 patients (10%); 6 of 11 (55%) patients with dyspnea received midazolam versus 12 of 175 (7%) patients with other indications ($p < 0.001$). Of the patients who received palliative sedation, 23% were discharged alive in contrast to 80% of the patients who did not receive palliative sedation ($p < 0.001$). Interestingly, propofol was included in the palliative sedation policy, mostly to be used in cases in which patients were refractory to midazolam, but this drug was never used.

Palliative sedation is a well-established intervention at the end of life in patients who are terminally ill, in whom death is imminent, and in whom suffering persists after maximization of standard medical treatments. Proportionality is crucial to the ethics of this practice, and consent should be obtained. Consultation with palliative care experts is highly recommended. Sedation should be started at the lowest possible dosage and titrated up until controlling the symptom.

TABLE 16.2. **Richmond Agitation Sedation Scale (RASS)**

Score	Term	Description
+4	Combative	Overtly combative, violent, immediate danger to staff
+3	Very agitated	Pulls or removes tube(s) or catheter(s); aggressive
+2	Agitated	Frequent non-purposeful movement, fights ventilator
+1	Restless	Anxious but movements not aggressive or vigorous
0	Alert and calm	
−1	Drowsy	Not fully alert, but has sustained awakening (eye opening/eye contact) to voice (≥10 sec)
−2	Light sedation	Briefly awakens with eye contact to voice (<10 sec)
−3	Moderate sedation	Movement or eye opening to voice (but no eye contact)
−4	Deep sedation	No response to voice, but movement or eye opening to physical stimulation
−5	Unarousable	No response to voice or physical stimulation

Procedure for RASS assessment

1.   Observe patient

    a. Patient is alert, restless, or agitated.   (score 0 to +4)

2.   If not alert, state patient's name and say to open eyes and look at speaker.

    b. Patient awakens with sustained eye opening and eye contact.   (score −1)

(continued)

TABLE 16.2. **Continued**

Score	Term	Description
	c. Patient awakens with eye opening and eye contact, but not sustained.	(score –2)
	d. Patient has any movement in response to voice but no eye contact.	(score –3)
3.	When no response to verbal stimulation, physically stimulate patient by shaking shoulder and/or rubbing sternum.	
	e. Patient has any movement to physical stimulation.	(score –4)
	f. Patient has no response to any stimulation.	(score –5)

From reference 5.

In our case, the option of palliative sedation was discussed with the patient and his family. All agreed to it. Risks and benefits were discussed, and informed consent was obtained. The patient was moved to the palliative care unit. A midazolam infusion was started, and the dose was titrated until the shortness of breath was controlled about 6 hours later. The patient was drowsy but was able to have sustained awakening to voice for a short period of time (RASS score –1). The following day he passed away with his family at bedside.

KEY POINTS TO REMEMBER

- Palliative sedation is an intervention used to manage refractory symptoms at the end of life in patients who are terminally ill.
- The most common situations in which palliative sedation is used are terminal agitated delirium, refractory shortness of breath, and intractable pain.

- Informed consent should be obtained before using palliative sedation.
- Midazolam is the most common medication used to achieve palliative sedation.
- The smallest effective dose of palliative sedation should be used to control symptoms.

Suggested

Beller EM, van Driel ML, McGregor L, Truong S, Mitchell G. Palliative pharmacological sedation for terminally ill adults. Cochrane Database Syst Rev. 2015;1(1):CD010206.

Maltoni M, Scarpi E, Rosati M, Derni S, Fabbri L, Martini F, Amadori D, Nanni O. Palliative sedation in end-of-life care and survival: a systematic review. J Clin Oncol. 2012;30(12):1378–83.

Elsayem A, Curry Iii E, Boohene J, Munsell MF, Calderon B, Hung F, Bruera E. Use of palliative sedation for intractable symptoms in the palliative care unit of a comprehensive cancer center. Support Care Cancer. 2009;17(1):53–9.

Further Reading

Bruera E. Palliative sedation: when and how? *J Clin Oncol*. 2012;30(12):1258–1259.

Clemens KE, Faust M, Bruera E. Update on combined modalities for the management of breathlessness. *Curr Opin Support Palliat Care*. 2012;6(2):163–167.

Kloke M, Cherny N; ESMO Guidelines Committee. Treatment of dyspnoea in advanced cancer patients: ESMO Clinical Practice Guidelines. *Ann Oncol*. 2015;26(supp 5):169–173.

Krakauer EL. Sedation at the end of life. In: Cherny NI, Fallon MT, Kaasa S, Portenoy RK, Currow DC, eds. *Oxford Textbook of Palliative Medicine*. Oxford University Press; 2018:1134–1141.

Raho JA. Palliative sedation: a review of the ethical debate. *Health Care Ethics USA*. 2014;22(3):15–23.

Twycross R. Reflections on palliative sedation. *Palliat Care*. 2019;12:1178224218823511.

References

1. Maltoni M, Scarpi E, Rosati M, et al. Palliative sedation in end-of-life care and survival: a systematic review. *J Clin Oncol*. 2012;30(12):1378–1383.
2. Beller EM, van Driel ML, McGregor L, Truong S, Mitchell G. Palliative pharmacological sedation for terminally ill adults. *Cochrane Database Syst Rev*. 2015;1(1):CD010206.

3. Elsayem A, Curry III E, Boohene J, et al. Use of palliative sedation for intractable symptoms in the palliative care unit of a comprehensive cancer center. *Support Care Cancer*. 2009;17(1):53–59.

4. Ripamonti C, Bruera E. Dyspnea: pathophysiology and assessment. *J Pain Symptom Manage*. 1997;13(4):220–232.

5. Sessler CN, Gosnell MS, Grap MJ, et al. The Richmond Agitation–Sedation Scale: validity and reliability in adult intensive care unit patients. *Am J Respir Crit Care Med*. 2002;166:1338–1344.

17 Sialorrhea in Amyotrophic Lateral Sclerosis

Mark B. Bromberg

A 67-year-old woman began having difficulties articulating words 6 months ago. Her speech disturbance progressed, and she could no longer be understood over the telephone, and recently her family needed her to repeat many words during direct conversations. About 3 months ago she noted the need to swallow multiple times between bites to clear her food. She has also noted reduced strength of her lower lip, and when she bends over saliva escapes onto her chin, and she always has a tissue at the ready to wipe her lips and prevent drooling. She consulted with her primary care physician, who sent her to a neurologist. A diagnosis of progressive bulbar palsy was made, but over the past month she has developed weakness of her right and then left-hand muscles and the diagnosis was changed to bulbar-onset amyotrophic lateral sclerosis (ALS).

What do I do now?

Sialorrhea is excess saliva in the mouth, beyond the lip margin. Normal saliva volume varies, and 1–1.5 quarts or liters are produced a day. Between meals, swallowing to clear baseline (unstimulated) levels of saliva occurs three or four times per minute, and frequently a swallow is necessary partway through a long sentence. Sialorrhea occurs when there is insufficient clearance of saliva, not excessive production. Saliva pools in the mouth, but patients also describe excess fluid in the larynx, which may be heard as gurgling in the throat. Sialorrhea is a very common problem in ALS, affecting most patients who have bulbar involvement, whether due to lower or upper motor neuron loss. Sialorrhea is socially disquieting and can markedly affect a patient's social interactions and quality of life. It frequently interferes with sleep and with use of noninvasive ventilation, and it can increase the risk of aspiration pneumonia. There are several causative factors: inefficient clearing of unstimulated saliva volume in the mouth due to lip and tongue weakness during the oral phase (lower motor neuron loss) of swallowing, and poor laryngeal clearance of saliva due to weakness and incoordination during the pharyngeal and laryngeal phases (upper motor neuron loss). Further, there is thick or stringy (mucinous) saliva in the mouth, but more problematically in the larynx, which is difficult to clear by swallowing or coughing (which may be inefficient due to diaphragm weakness). The cause of thick saliva is likely the accumulation of the protein elements (mucin) and reduced water component due to relative dehydration. Thick secretions may occur without sialorrhea and can also represent bronchial secretions. Sialorrhea is also common in Parkinson's disease and other neurodegenerative diseases, and in children with developmental conditions such as cerebral palsy.

Saliva is a complex fluid consisting of water to moisten dry food and consolidate the bolus during swallowing and proteins for oral health (protection, pH buffering, tooth integrity, antimicrobial action), and xerostomia (absence of saliva production) frequently leads to loss of teeth. Saliva is produced by three paired major glands (parotid, submandibular and sublingual glands) and also small minor glands. The major glands are encapsulated, while the minor glands are not and are distributed throughout the oral cavity. In the unstimulated state the parotid gland produces 20% of saliva, as well as the enzyme alpha-amylase (which breaks down starches). The submandibular gland produces 70% of saliva in the unstimulated state, as well as alpha-amylase and mucin (which acts as a lubricant [mucus]). The sublingual gland produces 10% of saliva, as well as mucin. Saliva volume increases fivefold in the stimulated state, and the increase is mostly from the parotid gland. Saliva production is mediated by reflex arcs with afferent limbs from chemoreceptors in taste buds and mechanoreceptors in periodontal ligaments (chewing) to the medulla, and efferent limbs mainly by the parasympathetic nervous system (mediated by acetylcholine) and less by the sympathetic nervous system (mediated by epinephrine). Activation of either nervous system increases saliva production; the cholinergic system produces serous saliva, and the adrenergic system produces mucin. There are also emotional factors, such as anticipating a "mouth-watering meal" or feeling fear and anxiety, resulting in a "cotton mouth."

There are four approaches to managing sialorrhea:

1. Hydration
2. Pharmacological manipulations to reduce saliva production (anticholinergic properties, beta-blockers, botulinum toxin)
3. Mechanical methods to physically remove saliva
4. Salivary gland destruction to reduce production.

Efficacy of treatment is difficult to assess as it is not possible to accurately measure saliva, and the degree of sialorrhea/amount of saliva can vary through the day. Perhaps the most meaningful estimation is by patient subjective report, but there are formal questionnaires, and two have been validated in ALS patients (Oral Secretion Scale and Sialorrhea Secretion Scale). Saliva production can be somewhat quantitated over a limited time duration (minutes) by placing dry cotton balls or gauze rolls in the mouth and weighing them after a set time.

Most drugs used for sialorrhea have different original indications and are selected in ALS for their anticholinergic side effects or beta-blockade effects. Only a few randomized controlled studies for these medications have been conducted in ALS patients, and efficacy studies are based on before-and-after-treatment comparisons and clinical experience. Treatment guidelines are available based on clinical practice habits, but the choice of drugs and the order of use are partially based on regional drug availability and cost.

PHARMACOLOGICAL MANIPULATION

Before pharmacological management, consideration should be given to overall hydration as many ALS patients have insufficient fluid intake, and dehydration leads to a reduced water component of saliva and an increased protein content (thicker saliva). Fluid needs can be calculated by nutritional formulas. The parasympathetic nerves are the main activator of salivary glands, mediated by acetylcholine at muscarinic receptors, and drugs that have anticholinergic effects (muscarinic antagonists) are most commonly used as first-line management. Some of the drugs have more than one use in ALS. Drugs that block beta-adrenergic receptors have been tried to a lesser extent in ALS to reduce secretion of mucus. Table 17.1 provides information about medications used to treat sialorrhea in patients with ALS.

TABLE 17.1. **Drugs Used to Treat Sialorrhea in ALS**

Drugs	Dose	Side Effects
Amitriptyline	12.5–50 mg PO HS	Drowsiness, constipation
Scopolamine	1 mg/72 hr patch	Drowsiness, skin irritation
Glycopyrrolate	1–2 mg PO QD–BID	Constipation
Atropine 1% ophthalmologic solution	1–2 gtts PRN	Bad taste
Oxybutynin	5 mg PO TID	Constipation
Propranolol	10 mg PO BID	
Metoprolol	25 mg PO BID	

BID = twice daily, gtts = drops, HS = at bedtime, PO = orally, PRN = as needed; QD = once a day, TID = three times a day.
Many drugs can be crushed and administered through a gastric feeding tube if the patient is unable to swallow.

First-Choice Medications

- Anticholinergic drugs
  - Amitriptyline: common first-choice drug; also effective for pseudobulbar affect, which affects ~30% of patients; improves sleep
  - Scopolamine (hyoscine): transdermal patch
  - Glycopyrrolate: primary indication for the reduction of saliva
  - Atropine: ophthalmologic drops under the tongue; used to "titrate" excess saliva
  - Oxybutynin: primary use is to reduce bladder urgency, which affects ~20% of patients
- Beta-blocker drugs
  - Propranolol and metoprolol
- Other drugs
  - Guaifenesin: reduces viscosity of tracheal secretions
  - Papain: proteolytic enzyme to break down protein in mucin

These drugs have 40–60% efficacy as rated by providers and show moderate efficacy in controlled trials in other diseases with sialorrhea. The most common side effect is a dry mouth from overtreatment, and the drug effect can cycle within a day from satisfactory control to insufficient saliva, but this is temporary as the drugs have short half-lives. Higher doses can cause constipation, and in the elderly, amitriptyline can cause drowsiness.

Second-Choice Medications

Botulinum toxin injections can be performed by a variety of providers, most commonly by neurologists who manage patients with ALS. Injections into the glands reduce the release of acetylcholine from presynaptic terminals, and are used when anticholinergic medications are not effective. The toxin binds irreversibly in nerve terminals, but nerve regeneration restores connectivity and the return of saliva production, and thus injections must be repeated ~3–6 months. Two strains of botulinum toxin, type A and B, have been used in ALS. There are several brand preparations for type A; all toxins have different dose units. Assessment and comparison of efficacy is difficult for the following reasons:

- A range of doses have been used.
- Different numbers of glands have been injected.

- The sites within glands and the number of sites injected differ.
- Injections have been either unguided or guided with ultrasound.
- A range of endpoint measures have been used.
- Some patients were refractory to anticholinergic medications yet some were continued on them.

From 12 studies using strain A, ~50% of patients had less saliva after injections; from three studies using strain B, 100% showed efficacy. For the positive trials, saliva reduction was noted between 3 and 12 weeks. Side effects were a dry mouth.

MECHANICAL METHODS

Oral suction devices are effective at removing saliva in the mouth but cannot reach thick secretions in the larynx. The suction pump is bulky and noisy. Frequent use of suction could possibly stimulate saliva production, resulting in a positive feedback loop. A cough-assist device can be used to help remove saliva in the larynx, including thick secretions. The device is a machine, more functionally called an "in-exsufflator," that augments a cough. A hose leads from a small portable box to a face mask. The machine augments the volume of air inhaled prior to a cough, and then creates a suction to help pull pulmonary secretions up and out with the exhalation phase.

SALIVARY GLAND IRRADIATION

External-beam radiation therapy is an option in patients who have not responded to anticholinergic medications or botulinum toxin. Treatment variables include source of radiation (protons, electrons), number of treatments, dose per treatment and total dose, dosing time period, and radiation field. A review of 10 studies indicated ~85% reduction in saliva compared to baseline, with improvement at a median time of 2 months (1–7 months). There was no difference between proton and electron beams, no indication of a dose–response (median dose 12 Gy, range 3–48 Gy), and no indication that larger fields or radiation were more effective. A small percentage of patients who received 15 Gy or less experienced a loss of efficacy over time. A dry mouth was experienced by 40% of patients, and 10%

experienced common symptoms of radiation in the form of mucositis and pain, taste change, and skin changes.

SURGICAL CONSIDERATIONS

Surgical procedures have been performed on patients with cerebral palsy and intractable sialorrhea, but not in ALS patients. A number of procedures include repositioning the salivary gland ducts.

CONCLUSION

It is important to query ALS patients about excess saliva even when it is not apparent clinically, as sialorrhea is socially distressing and affects the patient's quality of life. Anticholinergic medications have some efficacy in most patients, and some drugs are also effective for other ALS symptoms. Not all patients respond to their satisfaction, and botulinum toxin injections and salivary gland irradiation are additional options. Thick secretions are problematic to manage, and beta-blocking medications may be helpful.

KEY POINTS TO REMEMBER

- Sialorrhea is common in ALS patients with bulbar weakness, and efforts should be made to manage saliva production.
- Management is challenging and may not meet with full success.

Further Reading

Banfi P, Ticozzi N, Lax A, Guidugli GA, Nicolini A, Silani V. A review of options for treating sialorrhea in amyotrophic lateral sclerosis. *Respir Care.* 2015;60:446–454.

Bourry N, Guy N, Achard JL, Verrelle P, Clavelou P, Lapeyre M. Salivary glands radiotherapy to reduce sialorrhea in amyotrophic lateral sclerosis: dose and energy. *Cancer Radiother.* 2013;17:191–195.

McGeachan AJ, Hobson EV, Al-Chalabi A, et al. A multicentre evaluation of oropharyngeal secretion management practices in amyotrophic lateral sclerosis. *Amyotroph Lateral Scler Frontotemporal Degener.* 2017;18:1–9.

Squires N, Humberstone M, Wills A, Arthur A. The use of botulinum toxin injections to manage drooling in amyotrophic lateral sclerosis/motor neurone disease: a systematic review. *Dysphagia.* 2014;29:500–508.

18 Death Rattle

Margaret L. Campbell

Sheila has been transferred from the hospital to her home and is enrolled in hospice. She suffered an acute stroke, complicating her underlying dementia. On baseline assessment the hospice nurse notes hypotension, shallow breathing, and sounds of retained secretions. The nurse concludes that Sheila has no signs of distress but with hypotension and shallow breathing death is likely in hours to days. Sheila's daughter asks about the noisy breathing. She Googled it and saw the term "death rattle" used. She asks, "Is this something that needs to be treated? Is my mother suffering from this?"

What do I do now?

Death rattle is a condition that occurs naturally during the last hours of life, developing in about half of all patients.[1,2] It can be distressing for both professional caregivers and families of dying patients to hear. A death rattle is produced when the patient is near death and is too weak or hypersomnolent to clear or swallow pharyngeal secretions; even small volumes of secretions will produce sounds in the resonant pharyngeal space. Death rattle usually becomes audible 24 to 48 hours before death.

Conventionally, medications have been used to reduce or eliminate the patient noise and thus ease listeners' distress. However, topical, oral, or parenteral anticholinergic/antisecretory medications have often been associated with adverse effects such as dry mouth, urinary retention, visual disturbance, and confusion. These medications have included atropine, hyoscine glutamate, and glycopyrrolate.[2] Ironically, patients with a high anticholinergic drug load from prescribed medications were more likely to develop death rattle.[3] Attempts to remove the secretions by suctioning leads to adverse patient outcomes such as discomfort, bleeding, and vomiting.[4] Two systematic reviews concluded that there are no medication or nonmedication treatments that are superior to placebo.[5,6] Postural drainage by repositioning patients onto their side is a basic strategy that is largely without adverse patient outcomes and may be useful.

The general belief among healthcare professionals is that patients with death rattle are not experiencing distress. Conventional treatments are generally undertaken to appease family and staff, but these treatments may be more burdensome than beneficial to the patient. To date there have been no attempts to understand prescribing practices. Further, nonbeneficial treatments increase the cost of care.

While the efficacy of treatments for death rattle remains under investigation, the effect on the patient has been studied in only one prospective investigation.[1] Patients who were near death were stratified into those with and without death rattle. The patients were observed, and death rattle and respiratory distress were measured; there was no respiratory distress in either group. This was the first study to determine in a systematic fashion whether respiratory distress is associated with death rattle.

As predicted, this naturally occurring noisy sound at the end of life is not indicative of patient distress. It is, in fact, a signifier of impending death when there is an associated diminished consciousness such that normally swallowed or cleared secretions are retained in the pharynx. Sometimes, these noisy sounds become quite loud, paralleling the variance in other airway noises such as snoring. For example, snoring can be very subtle or loud enough to be heard at some distance from the sleeper.

It remains clinically counterproductive to prescribe medications with limited or no effectiveness in the face of *no* patient distress. Most of the medications routinely used to control pharyngeal secretions are anticholinergics that can induce urinary retention, dry mouth, and confusion, although we cannot be certain that the patient is able to experience them. Thus, with palliative care goals to minimize patient burden or harm, it stands to reason that medications and other interventions such as suctioning that have adverse effects and limited utility should be withheld. A better avenue to assuage family members' and clinicians' distress at hearing death rattle that does not entail medicating the patient is to normalize the sounds of death rattle for those who hear it.[7]

Changing routine practice entails a number of processes well described in evidence-based practice resources.[8] Novice clinicians new to the care of dying patients must have an evidence-based orientation. Thus, it is incumbent on educators to stay abreast of research findings that inform practice. The adage "we've always done it this way" has no place in an evidence-based clinical setting. The clinician who understands that death rattle does not require suctioning or medication will be equipped to help the family understand the noise and its significance.

Analogies are helpful to explain an unfamiliar phenomenon. Death rattle can be likened to snoring, which is a common, familiar sound. Since the small amounts of secretions make noise in the resonant tube (airway), another analogy is to compare the sound of death rattle to the noise made when chasing the last bit of liquid from the bottom of a glass with a straw.

We may want to acknowledge that dying can be a "messy" experience characterized by incontinence, odors, and sometimes noisy breathing. The mess, fuss, and noise associated with birth are not viewed negatively; in fact, they are normalized. Must we attempt to "sanitize" the noise that may occur during dying with medications? Can we normalize the sounds of death rattle for those who hear it?

CONCLUSIONS

Death rattle was not associated with respiratory distress among a sample of patients who were near death. In many cases, antisecretory agents did not produce quiet breathing—which begs the question about why they are still being used or at the very least why they are not discontinued when death rattle persists. There is no patient justification for the initiation of antisecretory medications. Interventions to assuage family or staff discomfort with death rattle remain to be identified.

The hospice nurse explained what produced the noise in Sheila's throat and that the sound was normal and not indicative of distress. She went on to explain that signs of distress, such as restlessness or rapid breathing, were not evident. She showed Sheila's daughter how to position her mother on her side with a towel under her face to catch any drooling saliva or secretions.

KEY POINTS TO REMEMBER

- Death rattle is common among patients in the last days before death.
- There is no patient distress, although listeners may be uncomfortable.
- Treating the patient with medication in the face of no distress is counterintuitive.
- Listener distress may be assuaged by teaching about the source of the noisy breathing and the absence of patient distress signs.

References

1. Campbell ML, Yarandi HN. Death rattle is not associated with patient respiratory distress: is pharmacologic treatment indicated? *J Palliat Med.* 2013;16(10):1255–1259.

2. Wildiers H, Dhaenekint C, Demeulenaere P, et al. Atropine, hyoscine butylbromide, or scopolamine are equally effective for the treatment of death rattle in terminal care. *J Pain Symptom Manage.* 2009;38(1):124–133.

3. Sheehan C, Clark K, Lam L, Chye R. A retrospective analysis of primary diagnosis, comorbidities, anticholinergic load, and other factors on

treatment for noisy respiratory secretions at the end of life. *J Palliat Med.* 2011;14(11):1211–1216.

4. Watanabe H, Taniguchi A, Yamamoto C, Odagiri T, Asai Y. Adverse events caused by aspiration implemented for death rattle in patients in the terminal stage of cancer: a retrospective observational study. *J Pain Symptom Manage.* 2018;56(1):e6–e8.

5. Kolb H, Snowden A, Stevens E. Systematic review and narrative summary: treatments for and risk factors associated with respiratory tract secretions (death rattle) in the dying adult. *J Adv Nurs.* 2018;74(7):1446–1462.

6. Wee B, Hillier R. Interventions for noisy breathing in patients near to death. *Cochrane Database Syst Rev.* 2008;1:CD005177.

7. Campbell ML. Assuaging listener distress from patient death rattle. *Ann Palliat Med.* 2019;8(supp 1):S58–S60.

8. Melnyk BM, Fineout-Overholt E. *Evidence-Based Practice in Nursing and Healthcare.* 2nd ed. Wolters Kluwer/Lippincott Williams and Wilkins; 2011.

Index

For the benefit of digital users, indexed terms that span two pages (e.g., 52–53) may, on occasion, appear on only one of those pages.

Note: Tables, figures, and boxes are indicated by *t*, *f*, and *b* following the page number

acute respiratory failure (ARF), 88, 89–91
advance care planning, 56–57
amyotrophic lateral sclerosis (ALS). *See* sialorrhea in amyotrophic lateral sclerosis
anxiety. *See* dyspnea/anxiety cycle
ascites, 51, 101–2
   diagnosis, 102–3
   etiology, 103
   symptoms, 102
   treatment, 103–7

benzodiazepines, 27–28
brain natriuretic peptide (BNP) levels, 52
Breathing, Thinking, Functioning (BTF) Model, 32*f,* 32–35, 42
breathing techniques, 25–26
breathlessness. *See* dyspnea/breathlessness
breathlessness services, 29
bronchopulmonary dysplasia (BPD), palliative care for infants with, 95–96
   primary palliative care in NICU, 96–98

cancer patients, dyspnea in. *See also* lung cancer; noninvasive ventilation
   reversible causes of and treatments for, 135–36, 137*t*
cardiac electrical device, interrogation of, 53
catheters, drainage, 106–7. *See also* tunneled pleural catheter
chemotherapy, 104
   hyperthermic intraperitoneal, 104
   systemic, 84
chest tube. *See* catheters; tunneled pleural catheter

chronic breathlessness syndrome, 40. *See also* dyspnea/breathlessness
chronic obstructive pulmonary disease. *See* COPD
cognitive-behavioral therapy, 44
congenital heart disease, dyspnea in pediatric, 61–63
   afterload reduction, 65
   fluid management, 63–64
controlled breathing, 25–26
COPD (chronic obstructive pulmonary disease)
   end stages of
      eligibility criteria for hospice enrollment, 120
      medications, 122
      nutrition, 120
      pacing activity, 120–21
      positioning, 121
      supplemental oxygen, 121–22
      toileting, 121
      trajectory of dyspnea at end of life, 122–23
   overview of, 22
   psychosocial needs of COPD patients, 23–24
   treatment of
      inhalation devices, 8–18
      inhaled medications, 9*t*
      reducing dyspnea by optimizing, 7–19
crackles, bibasilar, 51

death rattle, 153–56
dehydration, 112–13, 148
delirium, 115

dementia, panting for breath in end-stage, 109–10
  family guidance, 116
  pneumonia, 110
  symptom observation, 113–15
  treatment of, 113–15
    antibiotics vs. no antibiotics, 111–12
    food and fluids, 112–13
    medication review, 115–16
dietary sodium restriction, 55
distraction techniques, 44
diuresis, 53–54
diuretics, 104
double effect, principle of, 138
drainage catheters, 106–7. *See also* tunneled pleural catheter
dry powder inhalers (DPIs), 9*t*, 12*t*, 14–19, 15*f*
  advantages and disadvantages, 12*t*
  vs. nebulizers, 18
  Neohaler, 9*t*, 16*f*
Dyspnea-12, 3, 4*b*
dyspnea/anxiety cycle, 23, 24*f*
dyspnea/breathlessness, 22, 113. *See also specific topics*
  assessment tools
    multidimensional, 3–4
    unidimensional, 2, 3*f*
    observation scale, xi, 5–6
  defined, xi, 2, 113, 127–28
  overview and nature of, xi–xii, 2, 22
  physiology, 22–23
  terminology, xi
  treatment/management
    of acute episodes, 28
    breathlessness services, 29
    nonpharmacological, 21*b*–23*b*, 24–27, 65–66, 113
    pharmacological, 27–28, 66, 113–14
dyspnea crisis, 28
  defined, 28, 40
  steps for managing, 28

echocardiogram (ECHO), 52
edema, peripheral, 51
Edmonton Symptom Assessment Scale (ESAS), 71
ejection fraction (EF), 52
energy conservation techniques, 26–27
episodic dyspnea/breathlessness
  assessment of, 41
  preventing, 43–44
  treatment of, 42
    cognitive strategies, 44
    during an episode of breathlessness, 43
    pharmacological, 45
extubation. *See under* mechanical ventilation
exudative effusion, 78–79

fans, handheld, 26
fever, 114

Global Initiative for Chronic Obstructive Lung Disease (GOLD) guidelines, 8

heart failure (HF), episodic dyspnea in, 57
  assessment, 50–51
  diagnostics, 52–53
  etiology, 51–52
  preventing dyspnea recurrence, 55–56
    advance care planning, 56–57
    symptom and weight home monitoring, 56
    symptom management plans, 56
  progressive nature of HF, 66–67
  treatment of, 49*b*–55*b*, 53–55
    guideline-directed medical therapies (GDMTs), 54–55
    pharmacological, 53–55
    treating comorbid conditions, 55
heliox, 73
hospice enrollment, eligibility criteria for, 120
hydration, 112–13, 140, 147, 148. *See also* dehydration

hypersalivation. *See* sialorrhea in amyotrophic lateral sclerosis
hyperthermic intraperitoneal chemotherapy (HIPEC), 104
hypoplastic left heart syndrome (HLHS), 61, 63–64, 64*f*

inhalation devices, 8–18. *See also* dry powder inhalers; metered-dose inhalers; nebulizers; soft mist inhalers
advantages and disadvantages, 12*t*
inhaled medications, 9*t*
inhaler device training, 19
intraperitoneal hyperthermic chemotherapy, 104

jugular vein distention (JVD), 50

large-volume abdominal paracentesis (LVP), 105–6
lean-forward position, 25
lung cancer, chronic dyspnea in patients with, 69–74, 135. *See also* noninvasive ventilation

malignant pleural effusion (MPE), 78
diagnosis, 78–79
prognosis, 79
treatment options, 80–84, 83*t*
mechanical ventilation (MV). *See also* noninvasive ventilation
withdrawal of invasive, 125, 133
advance preparation for, 127
duration of survival after, 133
extubation considerations, 130–32
measuring distress during, 127–28, 129*t*
oxygen following, 132–33
premedication for anticipated distress, 128–30
sample rapid wean, 131*t*
weaning method, 130

metered-dose inhalers (MDIs), 9*t*, 12*t*, 13–18, 14*f*, 122
advantages and disadvantages, 12*t*
vs. nebulizers, 18
overview and nature of, 8–13
vs. SMIs, 17
Modified Medical Research Council (MMRC) dyspnea scale, 4
morphine, 73, 113–14, 122, 131*t*, 133
Multidimensional Profile (MDP), 3–4

nebulizers, 18
advantages and disadvantages, 12*t*
neuromuscular blocking agents (NMBAs), 127
neuropsychiatric symptoms, 115
noninvasive ventilation (NIV), treating dyspnea in lung cancer with, 87–91

opioid therapy, 45, 66, 113–15, 128–29. *See also* morphine
systemic, 27, 73
Organ Procurement Organization (OPO), 127
orthopnea, 50
oxygen, supplemental, 121–22, 132–33

pain, 114–15
palliative sedation, 136–42
defined, 136
medications used for, 139, 139*b*
paracentesis, 105–6
peritoneovenous shunts (PVSs), 103, 105
physical activity, 25
pleurodesis, 81–82
pneumonia, 110, 111*t*
positioning, 25–26
potassium, 52
pulmonary rehabilitation (PR), 25
pursed-lip breathing, 25–26

recovery breathing, 26
relaxation, 44
renal function, 52

respiratory distress. *See* dyspnea/breathlessness
Respiratory Distress Observation Scale
    (RDOS), 4–5, 5*b*, 128, 129*t*, 131*t*
respiratory distress syndrome (RDS), 96
respiratory failure. *See* acute respiratory
    failure
Richmond Agitation Sedation Scale
    (RASS), 139–40, 141*t*

saliva, 146–47. *See also* sialorrhea in
    amyotrophic lateral sclerosis
serum–ascites albumin gradient (SAAG), 103
shortness of breath. *See* dyspnea/
    breathlessness
shunts, vascular, 103, 105
sialorrhea in amyotrophic lateral sclerosis
    (ALS), 145–48, 151
  drugs used to treat, 148*t*, 148
  mechanical methods, 150
  pharmacological manipulation, 148
    first-choice medications, 149
    second-choice medications, 149–50
  salivary gland irradiation, 150–51
  surgical considerations, 151

sodium restriction, 55
soft mist inhalers (SMIs), 9*t*, 17*f*
  advantages and disadvantages, 12*t*
  overview and nature of, 17

terminal extubation, 130. *See also*
    mechanical ventilation
terminal weaning, 130
  rapid, 130, 133 (*see also* mechanical
    ventilation)
thoracentesis, 80–81
toileting, 121
transjugular intrahepatic portosystemic
    shunt (TIPS), 105
tumor debulking, 104
tunneled pleural catheter (TPC), 81–82

vascular endothelial growth factor
    (VEGF), 104
ventilation. *See* noninvasive ventilation

weight gain, 51

x-ray, chest, 52